The Institute of Biology's
Studies in Biology

Introductory
Statistics
for Biology

Second Edition

R. E. Parker
B.Sc.

Senior Lecturer in Botany,
The Queen's University of Belfast

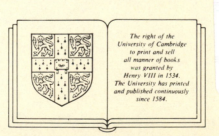

The right of the
University of Cambridge
to print and sell
all manner of books
was granted by
Henry VIII in 1534.
The University has printed
and published continuously
since 1584.

CAMBRIDGE UNIVERSITY PRESS

CAMBRIDGE

NEW YORK   PORT CHESTER

MELBOURNE   SYDNEY

Published by the Press Syndicate of the University of Cambridge
The Pitt Building, Trumpington Street, Cambridge CB2 1RP
40 West 20th Street, New York, NY 10011–4211, USA
10 Stamford Road, Oakleigh, Victoria 3166, Australia

First published by Edward Arnold 1973
Second edition published by Edward Arnold 1979
First published by Cambridge University Press 1991

Printed in Great Britain at the University Press, Cambridge

British Library cataloguing in publication data

Parker, Reginald Ernest
  Introductory statistics for biology.—2nd ed.
  —(Institute of Biology. Studies in biology:
  no. 43).
  1. Biometry
  I. Title   II. Series
  519.5′02′4574   QH323.5

ISBN 0 521 42778 9 paperback

Printed and bound in Great Britain by
Hartnolls Limited, Bodmin, Cornwall

General Preface to the Series

Recent advances in biology have made it increasingly difficult for both students and teachers to keep abreast of all the new developments in so wide-ranging a subject. The New Studies in Biology, are published to facilitate resolution of this problem. Each text provides a synthesis of a field and gives the reader an authoritative overview of the subject without unnecessary detail.

The Studies series originated 20 years ago but its vigour has been maintained by the regular production of new editions and the introduction of additional titles as new themes become clearly identified. It is appropriate for the New Studies in their refined format to appear at a time when the public at large has become conscious of the beneficial application of knowledge from the whole spectrum from molecular to environmental biology. The new series is set to provide a great boon to the new generation of students as the original series did to their fathers.

1986

Institute of Biology
20 Queensberry Place
London SW7 2DZ

Contents

How to Use this Book

Statistics is not presented here as a branch of mathematics but as a logical commonsense development from very simple beginnings. The difficulties, such as they are, do not lie in mathematical manipulation but in grasping a few simple but unfamiliar concepts. Learning to apply statistical methods is rather like learning to swim or drive a car. One does not become fully proficient immediately and certainly not by just reading and thinking about it. Practical experience is all important. Through practical experience one acquires practical skills and real understanding.

Do not wait until you have some numerical data to analyse before turning to this book. Start now, at the beginning, and try to understand why biologists need to think in terms of statistics and to employ statistical methods. Then, whether you are convinced or not, work steadily on through the book. Master each section as you go, attempt *all* the problems at the ends of the chapters, and check your numerical solutions and logical conclusions with the solutions provided. You will not regret making the effort: the understanding and skill that you acquire will be of lasting value to you, both in your biological work and outside.

Belfast 1978   R. E. P.

1 Probability and Statistics

1.1 Why statistics?

The first problem that most students of biology have with statistics is in understanding why they need to study the subject at all. It is possible, during the first few years of biology at school, to learn a great deal about animals, plants and biological systems in terms of discoveries made by biologists *in the past*. It takes more than this, however, to make a real biologist. A biologist must understand how biological knowledge has been obtained and is being constantly modified and extended by research. It is here that an appreciation of the role of statistics becomes meaningful. For a biologist aiming to make his or her own contribution to biological knowledge some understanding of statistics is essential.

An appreciation of the role of statistics in biology comes most easily through personal involvement in biological investigation, hence the importance of project work, provided that its objective is to discover something new. In part, the role of statistics is direct, enabling us to make statements and draw conclusions of scientific significance from the limited evidence we have obtained by the examination of one or more relatively small samples. For example, suppose as part of a study of the effect of geographical isolation we wish to make statements about the body measurements of the population of field mice on a certain island. We could never hope to catch all of the mice, there might be many thousands, so we trap a sample of them (perhaps 50) and measure this representative group. But when reporting our finding of, for example, 'mean tail length', we would want this to relate to the population as a whole and not just to our small sample. We could do this by using *confidence limits* (see Chapter 2).

Again, suppose that we wished to compare two 'wetting agents' as additions to foliar fertilizers. In our experiment we would only be able to treat a limited number of, for example, lettuce plants, but our conclusions would need to apply to all lettuces of the particular variety used in the experiment. Before concluding that there was no real difference between the wetting agents or that one was more effective than the other we would be likely to need a *test of significance* (see § 1.4 and Chapter 3).

Another role of statistics lies in the simplification of data with the detection and definition of trends or relationships. In biology observed relationships are rarely clear-cut. Even when an underlying relationship is simple our picture of it is often confused by uncontrolled variation. This role can be seen in a simple form in Chapter 8, where the linear component of the relationship between temperature (°C) and water-loss (mg) of a group of mice is extracted and defined by means of *linear regression*. With advances in techniques of environmental sensing, and in the recording and processing of data, the role of statistics in simplification and extraction of trends is increasing. Even when a computer is used for the data processing it must be programmed with the appropriate statistical instructions. The use of statistical methods as tools in biology has had several important repercussions. The introduction of new physical and chemical methods, such as the electron microscope, radioisotopes, and chromatography, led to the opening up of new fields of biological enquiry. The same is true of statistics: there are branches of biology which only became possible with the development of the necessary statistical tools, for example, quantitative population genetics. More generally, advances in the design of biological surveys and experiments have come about as a direct result of development in statistical techniques. The close relationship between experimental design and data analysis is discussed in Chapters 9 and 10.

1.2   Probability

Whenever we draw conclusions relating to whole populations from the evidence of samples, for example, when we fit confidence limits or make tests of significance, these conclusions are always couched in terms of probability. In statistics *probability* takes on a full quantitative meaning, having values ranging from zero which is equivalent to impossibility, to unity which is equivalent to complete certainty. There are two ways of estimating the probability of a particular kind of outcome: one, *a priori*, is from some knowledge of the underlying process, or at least some hypothesis concerning it, e.g. for a cross between a heterozygote (Gg) and a homozygote (gg) we can estimate the probability of a single random offspring being (Gg) as 0.5, the same as its being (gg). The other way, *empirical*, is by observation of the outcome of a number of actual trials, thus:

$$\text{estimated probability, } p = \frac{\text{number of successes}}{\text{number of trials}}$$

where a 'success' is the kind of outcome in which we are interested. For example, the probability of a seed, taken at random from a population, being capable of germination may be estimated by carrying out a germination test on a sample of seeds from that population. The results of such a test are conventionally expressed in the form of a percentage (i.e. $100 \times p$). In general, the larger the sample examined the more closely will the estimated probability approximate to the true one.

In order to find out why observations tend to fall into classes with the frequencies they do, we compare the *observed* frequencies with the frequencies which would be *expected* on the basis of a particular hypothesis. To obtain an expected frequency we simply multiply the expected probability by the total number of trials. For example, if we wished to discover whether two dominant genes were linked we could backcross double heterozygotes (AaBb) with double recessives (aabb) and count the number of organisms in each of the four phenotype classes. If the genes segregate independently (i.e. if there is no linkage) the expected probability for each class is the same and equal to 0.25. If we have a total of 400 offspring the expected frequency of each class would be $400 \times 0.25 = 100$. Note that every individual *must* belong to one of the four classes and that with equal probability of it falling in each one we partition the total probability of 1.0 into four equal parts of 0.25. (If we had chosen to make the $F_1 \times F_1$ cross the partition would have been into: 9/16, 3/16, 3/16, and 1/16.)

1.3   Probability distribution

In partitioning the total probability of 1.0 into several components, each corresponding to a different kind of outcome, we are exposing a simple probability distribution. We need to look more thoroughly into this because the distribution of probability is the key to a great deal of statistics. Let us begin with the simplest kind of situation, one in which at a single trial there are only two kinds of outcome.

Suppose that in an investigation of the relationship between a certain beetle species and its environment we wish to test the hypothesis that its known sensitivity to humidity is located in its antennae. We could take a beetle, remove its antennae, and place it in a choice-chamber where two different levels of humidity were maintained. If our hypothesis is true the probability of beetle choosing the high humidity is the same as the probability of its choosing the low, and is equal to 0.5. Provided that the choice-chamber was of suitable design two beetles could be introduced at the same time. What would the probability distribution be now? There are three different possible types of outcome: both move to high humidity, both move to low humidity, or one moves to high and the other to low. The corresponding probabilities are given in the table on p. 4.

Note that the probability of both beetles behaving in the same way is the *product* of the individual probabilities, as two conditions must be fulfilled before the outcome is attained. Also note that the probability of a mixed outcome is the *sum* of the probabilities of the different ways in which the same outcome can be attained. The table also shows the possible types of outcome and their probabilities for groups of three and four beetles. In this simple example the expected probabilities can be

Number of beetles	Possible outcomes				Number of possibilities
1	$H(\frac{1}{2})$			$L(\frac{1}{2})$	2
2	$HH(1/4)$		$\begin{matrix}HL\\LH\end{matrix}(\frac{1}{2})$	$LL(1/4)$	3
3	$HHH(1/8)$	$\begin{matrix}HHL\\HLH\\LHH\end{matrix}(3/8)$	$\begin{matrix}HLL\\LHL\\LLH\end{matrix}(3/8)$	$LLL(1/8)$	4
4	$HHHH\ (1/16)$	$\begin{matrix}HHHL\\HHLH\\HLHH\\LHHH\end{matrix}(1/4)$	$\begin{matrix}HHLL\\HLHL\\HLLH\\LHHL\\LHLH\\LLHH\end{matrix}(3/8)$	$\begin{matrix}HLLL\\LHLL\\LLHL\\LLLH\end{matrix}(1/4)$ $LLLL(1/16)$	5

easily worked out from first principles. More generally we compute the probabilities by expanding the expression $(p + q)^n$ where p is the probability of an individual, taken at random, falling into one of the two mutually exclusive catagories, $q = 1 - p$ (i.e. the probability of its falling into the other), and n is the number of individuals in the group. For $n = 4$ this gives:

$$(p + q)^4 = p^4 + 4p^3 q + 6p^2 q^2 + 4pq^3 + q^4$$

You may recognize this as the binomial expansion. The distribution of probability is discontinuous because however large the group (n) there will always be a finite number $(n + 1)$ of categories. In the present example the distribution is symmetrical. This is because $p = 0.5 = q$. More generally $p \neq 0.5$ and the distribution is asymmetrical.

1.4   Tests of significance

Suppose that we have conducted an experiment in which we placed eight beetles from which the antennae had been removed in a choice-chamber with high and low humidity compartments, and that all eight had moved to high humidity. What would we conclude? With such an extreme result we would probably be left in no doubt that the beetles were still sensitive to humidity differences and that our hypothesis should be rejected. But first examine Fig. 1–1 which represents in the form of a histogram* the probability distribution corresponding to $(p + q)^8$ where $p = 0.5 = q$. You will see that the outcome with the

* Conventionally such discontinuous distributions are represented by bar charts. Histograms are used here to emphasize the similarity between discontinuous distributions and continuous distributions to be met with later.

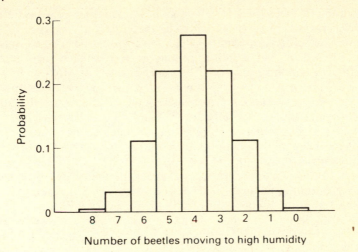

Fig. 1–1 Probabilities of different numbers of beetles, from 8 to 0, moving to high humidity: $p = 0.5$.

highest probability, the *expected* outcome, is the one with equal numbers of beetles moving to high and low humidity. The observed result, if the beetles are insensitive to humidity (i.e. if $p = q$), has a probability of $p^8 = 1/256$ (c. 0.004). We have therefore *either* to retain our hypothesis and accept that a very unlikely event has occurred *or* to reject our hypothesis and replace it with one in which $p > 0.5$. With such a low probability we would normally modify our hypothesis and conclude that the beetles were still sensitive to humidity differences, even with antennae removed.

The test consists of the computation of a probability corresponding to the result observed on the assumption of a particular hypothesis. If the probability is low (conventionally $\leqslant 0.05$) we conclude that the hypothesis is incorrect. If the probability is high (conventionally > 0.05) we conclude that the departure from expectation is not great enough for the hypothesis to be rejected. In general, it is necessary to take into account other possible outcomes which depart an equal or greater amount from expectation. In the above example there is only one other outcome with as great a departure, i.e. eight beetles moving to low humidity. We do not need to take account of this because intact beetles are known to move to *high* humidities and so the possibility of the opposite kind of behaviour does not arise. We are making what is known as a 'one-tailed' test (see also § 4.4).

It might be argued that in the example above we had no need of statistics because the conclusion was self-evident. Results are not always as extreme. Suppose that only six beetles had moved to high humidity the remaining two moving to low. It could be argued that as the beetles have shown a marked preference for high humidity they must still be sensitive to humidity differences and our hypothesis should be rejected. It might also be argued that as some beetles moved in each direction our hypothesis should be retained. This is just the sort of situation in which statistics can help. If we again turn to Fig. 1–1 we see that the probability corresponding to the observed result is now much greater. It is in fact $28p^6q^2 = 28/256 = 0.1094$. Before making the test, however, we must take into account the two more extreme results, i.e. of seven and eight beetles moving to high humidity. The total probability of the three types of outcome is $28/256 + 8/256 + 1/256 = 0.1445$ (c. 1/7).* This is well in excess of 0.05 (1/20) and so we would regard the observed departure from expectation as *not significant* and retain the hypothesis that the beetles have been rendered insensitive to humidity differences. In fact, tests of this kind, if repeated, would be expected, on average, to give as large or larger departure one in seven times, even though the beetles had been rendered insensitive.

In this first chapter we have become acquainted with the ways in which probability can be treated quantitatively, in particular how it can be partitioned to yield discontinuous probability distributions. We have also seen how we can use such a distribution in making tests of significance. Discontinuous distributions are related to observations of discrete events. Such observations are of great importance in biology and we will be examining the methods for their analysis in some detail in Chapters 4 to 7. In Chapters 2 and 3 we will direct our attention to observations which take the form of measurements on a continuous scale. The probability distributions of such measurements are continuous and this presents us with rather different problems and opportunities for analysis.

Problems

1–1 In a choice-chamber experiment like the one examined above what is the smallest number of beetles that could be used in an experiment and still give a significant result in a 'one-tailed' test?

1–2 A reasonable *a priori* probability of a child, taken at random, being a boy is 0.5, this being consistent with equal numbers of male and female sex chromosomes on gametogenesis in the male parent. How large a family, consisting of children of the same sex, would a biologist need to have before rejecting the general hypothesis of $p_{boy} = 0.5 = p_{girl}$ as applicable to his or her own relationship? (Assume the conventional significance level of 0.05.)

* This is, of course, again a 'one-tailed' test.

2 Continuous Distributions: Confidence Limits

2.1 A population represented by a sample

The populations about which we wish to make statements and draw conclusions are represented in biological surveys and experiments by samples (see § 1.1). These samples consist of individuals. In some investigations these individuals are whole plants or animals but more generally they range from individual cells, or even organelles, to plots of forest trees. They can take the form of organs, tissue preparations, extracts, and even environmental locations. Despite this diversity they have in common the fact that they contribute an item of information relating to one or more of their attributes. For the moment we are concerned only with situations in which there is information relating to one kind of attribute and in which the information consists of measurements on a continuous scale, such as weight, volume, area, length, concentration, rate, pH, etc.

Suppose that as part of an autecological study of the bracken fern (*Pteridium aquilinum*) we wished to assess the performance of the fern within a certain area, Area 1. Frond (leaf) length could be included among the performance parameters. There are thousands of fronds in the population of the area and they vary conspicuously in length. We might decide to measure a sample of 100 fronds. Clearly the sample should be representative and must therefore be selected without bias. This is more difficult to achieve than it might appear, simply measuring one frond here and another there in an irregular manner will not do. Ideally we should take a *random* sample but we will leave this problem for now and assume that the lengths of 100 fronds have been measured. The 100 measurements are added together and divided by the number of fronds (100) to obtain an average or mean length. This is a *sample mean* and it is our best estimate of the *population mean*. A simple statement of our sample mean, with the unstated implication that the population mean is likely to be rather similar, is not likely to be very satisfactory when we come to make comparisons between different areas and try to draw meaningful conclusions. We need to assess and state in some way the reliability of our sample mean as an estimate of the population mean. We can do this by attaching confidence limits.

2.2 The normal distribution

Clearly the reliability of a sample mean is bound up with the variability of the individual measurements and with the number of them that we have to average. We need then some measure of variability. The measure that we use is related in an important way to the kind of probability distribution shown by the individual measurements. For-tunately there is a strong tendency for the measurements of individuals in different populations to show the same kind of distribution, the *normal distribution*.

If we had measurements for a large number (for example 1000) of individuals in a population, e.g. frond length as in our example, we could group the measurements into size classes, count the number falling into each size class, and plot a frequency histogram to show how the individual measurements were distributed. (NB Measurements fall automatically into size classes if they are made to a certain degree of precision only.) As probability is the ratio of frequency to the total number of measurements (see § 1.2) the frequency histogram could be rescaled to illustrate the corresponding probability distribution. It would now indicate the distribution of probability of an individual measurement, taken at random, falling into each size class. The histogram produced is likely to be more or less symmetrical and to have a bell-like outline. In some respects it would resemble the histogram for a symmetrical binomial distribution, (Fig. 1–1), but would differ from this in two important respects. The range of a binomial distribution is fixed by the number of events recorded in each trial but the range of the population of measurements is not limited in this way. The number of classes in the binomial distribution is also fixed, $(n + 1)$, and the distribution of probability essentially discontinuous. We could not read from Fig. 1–1 the probability of $5\frac{1}{2}$ beetles moving to high and $2\frac{1}{2}$ beetles moving to low humidity. On the other hand, by making measurements to a high degree of precision and making enough of them a histogram could be prepared with a very large number of very narrow size classes and an outline that would approach closely a smooth curve. The theoretical curve towards which many natural probability distributions tend is called the *normal curve*.

2.3 Mean and standard deviation

Clearly the normal distribution cannot be defined in the same terms as a binomial distribution. The normal curve is defined by the expression:

$$Y = \frac{1}{\sigma \sqrt{(2\pi)}} e^{-[(X - \mu)^2/2\sigma^2]}$$

Fortunately we can use the properties of the normal distribution without using this expression but there are several important points to note about it. The variables X and Y are related through two parameters μ and σ. μ is the *mean*, the point about which the distribution is symmetrical, and σ is the *standard deviation*, a measure of the variability or spread of the measurements about the mean. The important point is that a normal distribution is completely defined by these two parameters; the other two quantities π and e are, of course, constants. Thus, if we know the standard deviation of a population we have the key to the distribution of probability about its mean. In practice we rarely know the population standard deviation, σ, but have to estimate it as s from the sample measurements. We can estimate σ as $s = \sqrt{[\Sigma(X - \overline{X})^2/(N-1)]}$, where the numerator is the sum of the squares of the deviations of X from its mean, and the denominator is one less than the number of measurements. You may wonder why the denominator is not N. If we knew the population mean (μ) the correct denominator would be N, but in practice we have to estimate μ as $\overline{X}$. If we have N values of X and compute $\overline{X} = \Sigma X/N$, then we have only $(N-1)$ values of X which are independent of $\overline{X}$, in other words we have only $(N-1)$ *degrees of freedom*. Having determined $\overline{X}$ the Nth value of X is also fixed. The above formula is rarely used to evaluate s because to do so is unnecessarily laborious and usually introduces rounding errors. Instead we use the algebraically equivalent expression:

$$s = \sqrt{\left(\frac{\Sigma X^2 - \dfrac{(\Sigma X)^2}{N}}{N-1} \right)}$$

NB ΣX^2 denotes the sum of the squares of all values of X taken singly, and $(\Sigma X)^2$ denotes the square of the sum of all values of X. The quantity $\Sigma(X - \overline{X})^2 \equiv \Sigma X^2 - ((\Sigma X)^2/N)$ is so often met with that it is referred to as the *sum-of-squares of* X and is denoted by Σx^2.

We have already seen in section 1.4 that given a hypothetical probability (p) and a group size (n) we can compute the terms of the corresponding binomial distribution and draw a histogram illustrating the probability distribution. From this histogram we can read off the probabilities of different kinds of outcome in terms of the heights or areas of the corresponding rectangle or rectangles. Figure 2–1 shows the probabilities of the seven different kinds of family composition for a family of six children, assuming $p_{boy} = 0.5 = p_{girl}$. The probability of a family including one or two boys is indicated by the total area of the two shaded rectangles. Now, in much the same way, the probability of an individual measurement, taken at random, falling between two stated values of X is given by the area of the figure bounded by the appropriate normal curve and the X axis, and lying between the verticals corresponding to the two X values. Figure 2–2 shows the probability distribution for heights of adult human males in a population. The probability of a man,

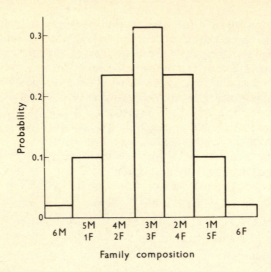

Fig. 2-1 Probabilities of the 7 different kinds of family composition for a family of 6 children: $p_{male} = p_{female} = 0.5$. The probability of a family including 1 or 2 boys is indicated by the area of the two shaded rectangles.

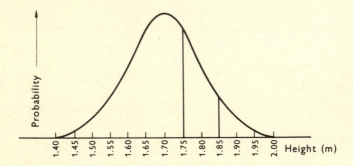

Fig. 2-2 Probability distribution for the heights of human adult males in a population. The probability of a single individual taken at random having a height falling between 1.75 m and 1.85 m is indicated by the area of the shaded part of the figure.

taken at random, having a height between 1.75 and 1.85 m is indicated by the area of the shaded part of the figure.

The shape of a particular normal curve, and therefore the corresponding distribution of probability, depends entirely on the standard deviation of the normal distribution which it represents. It is possible therefore to draw up tables for the areas beneath the curve (in terms of probability) between certain limiting values of X, provided that such values are expressed in terms of standard deviation units. Such tables are then true for all normal distributions. For example, we can read from such tables that the area between the line of symmetry (at $X = \mu$) and the line at one standard deviation above ($\mu + \sigma$) *or* below ($\mu - \sigma$) corresponds to a probability of 0.3413. Thus we can say that there is a probability of 0.6826 of a single value, taken at random, falling within one standard deviation of the mean. Similarly, a single value has a probability of 0.95 of falling within 1.96σ of the mean. In terms of frequency this means that 68.26% of all values lie between the limits $\mu \pm \sigma$ and 95% of all values lie between the limits $\mu \pm 1.96\sigma$ (Fig. 2–3). The probability that an individual value, taken at random, would fall within this range is 0.95: conversely given an individual value we can say that the probability of the true mean falling within 1.96σ of *it* must also be 0.95. It might appear at first sight that we have here a way of describing the reliability of a single random observation in estimating the population mean. Our estimate of the mean would be the single measurement and there would be a probability of 0.95 of the population mean lying within $\pm 1,96\sigma$ of it. The snag, of

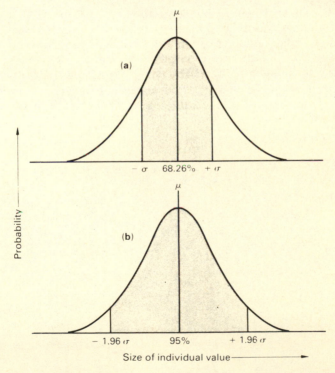

Fig. 2–3 Probability limits for the normal distribution defined in terms of standard deviation (σ): **(a)** 68.26% and **(b)** 95%.

course, is that a whole series of measurements would be needed for the estimation of the standard deviation.

2.4   Standard error of the mean and confidence limits

If a series of measurements were available we would use their mean to indicate the population mean rather than rely on a single measurement to do so. If a sample mean is to be used in this way we would need to know something about the distribution of sample means. We have seen that if we take a very large sample of measurements from a population, divide it into a series of small size classes and plot a frequency histogram, the outline of the histogram approaches a normal curve. If we were now to take these measurements in random groups (of N), calculate the means of these groups and prepare a frequency histogram from these, its outline would again approach a normal curve but one with less spread, i.e. with a smaller standard deviation (Fig. 2–4). It may be shown that the standard deviation of the means of N measurements from a population with a standard deviation of σ is $\sigma/\sqrt{N}$. Conventionally the standard deviation of a mean is known as its *standard error*. In the same way that we could use the standard deviation to describe the reliability of a single random measurement in indicating the population mean so we can use the standard error to indicate the reliability of a sample mean in doing so. Thus, having computed $\overline{X}$ (as $\Sigma X/N$) we can state that this is our best estimate of the true mean (μ) and attach *confidence limits* at a chosen level

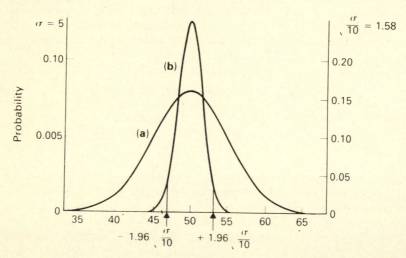

Fig. 2 4   Normal curves (a) for individual values of X with $\mu = 50$ and $\sigma = 5$, and (b) for means of ten values. 95% probability limits for means of 10 values.

of probability. For example, for the 0.95 level of probability we would compute $\overline{X} \pm 1.96\, s/\sqrt{N}$. The true mean then has a probability of 0.95 of falling within these limits, and conversely a probability of 0.05 of falling outside.

The probability level of 0.95 used in this example is conventionally employed in much biological work, such limits being known as *95% confidence limits*. Sometimes confidence limits at a different probability level are required and for this purpose another multiplier which will provide the appropriate partition of probability must be selected, e.g. for a probability of 0.99, giving 99% confidence limits, the multiplier is 2.576 because for a normal distribution 99% of the observations lie between $\mu \pm 2.576\sigma$. The general name for these multipliers is 'standardized normal deviate' or '*d*', and tables are available that give values of d for a series of probability levels. The probability values in such tables are conventionally given for total probability *outside* the limits (i.e. for the two 'tails' of the distribution): thus 1.96 is listed against $P = 0.05$ and 2.576 against $P = 0.01$.

In the same way that we do not know μ (population mean) but must estimate it as $\overline{X}$ (sample mean) so we do not know σ (population standard deviation) but must estimate it as s (sample standard deviation). However, provided that we have a relatively large number of measurements (e.g. $N > 30$) s approximates σ closely and the tabulated values of d may be used as indicated above, but see also section 2.5. The development of the above method for attaching confidence limits to means is based on the assumption that the individual measurements are normally distributed. It is a comforting fact that even when the individual measurements deviate from normality the sample means still tend to be normally distributed, provided that the samples are not too small.

Values of d for a series of probability levels, P

P	0.1	0.05	0.02	0.01	0.001	0.0001	0.00001
d	1.645	1.960	2.326	2.576	3.291	3.891	4.417

Let us now return to the problem of attaching confidence limits to the mean of our sample of 100 bracken frond lengths. When dealing with a large sample it is often a good idea to collect the data by tallying the numbers of measurements which fall into each of a series of size classes. Then instead of adding each value of X and X^2 separately we count the number of measurements in each size class, compute the contribution to ΣX and ΣX^2 by each size class and then sum these.

Completed tally sheet for sample of 100 bracken frond lengths.

Size class (mid pt)	*Tally*	*Frequency*	*Class × frequency*	*Class² × frequency*
0.7	1	1	0.7	0.49
0.8	𝍸 11	7	5.6	4.48
0.9	𝍸 𝍸 1	11	9.9	8.91
1.0	𝍸 𝍸 𝍸 𝍸 1	21	21.0	21.00
1.1	𝍸 𝍸 𝍸 𝍸 𝍸 1	26	28.6	31.46
1.2	𝍸 𝍸 𝍸 1111	19	22.8	27.36
1.3	𝍸 111	8	10.4	13.52
1.4	𝍸	5	7.0	9.80
1.5	11	2	3.0	4.50

$N = 100 \quad \Sigma X = 109.0 \quad \Sigma X^2 = 121.52$

NB The fronds were measured in m, to the nearest 0.1 m.

We estimate μ by $\bar{X} = \Sigma X/N = 109.0/100 = \underline{1.090 \text{ m}}$

We estimate σ by

$$s = \sqrt{\left(\frac{\Sigma X^2 - \frac{(\Sigma X)^2}{N}}{N-1}\right)} = \sqrt{\left(\frac{121.52 - \frac{109.0^2}{100}}{99}\right)} = 0.165\,45 \text{ m}$$

We compute standard error of the mean $= 0.16545/\sqrt{100}$
$= 0.016545$ m

95% confidence limits of μ are $1.090 \pm 1.96 \times 0.0165\,45$ m

i.e. $\underline{1.090 \pm 0.032}$ (1.058 to 1.122) m

Our best estimate of the mean frond length for the bracken population in Area 1 is 1.09 m, and taking account of both the variation between the individual fronds and the number of fronds measured we estimate that there is a probability of 0.95 that the mean of the whole population lies within the range 1.058 m to 1.122 m.

2.5 Confidence limits for the means of small samples

When using tabulated values of d it is important to remember that they refer to the relationship between probability and the deviation from the mean in units based on the true standard deviation (σ). In the estimation of σ by s there is always an element of approximation and hence uncertainty. What we need are multipliers based on deviation/$s_{\bar{X}}$ rather than deviation/$\sigma_{\bar{X}}$. This problem was solved in 1908 by William S.

Gosset an amateur statistician employed at Guinness' Brewery. He published under the name of 'Student' and provided us with tables of the required statistic t. In simple terms, the probabilities read from the table of t include an allowance for the uncertainty associated with the estimation of population standard deviation from a limited sample. For any particular level of probability t will have a greater value than the corresponding value of d, the difference depending on the size of sample used to compute s, or more precisely the number of degrees of freedom $(N - 1)$. Turn to the table on page 116 and note that for a particular probability level (say 0.05) t for ∞ degrees of freedom is the same as d, but as the number of degrees of freedom decreases t increases. The statistic t then provides us with a more general method for attaching confidence limits, applicable to both large and small samples. We compute the confidence limits as: $\overline{X} \pm t \times s/\sqrt{N}$, where the value of t used is read from the tables at the selected probability level (e.g. 95%) and for $(N - 1)$ degrees of freedom.

In an experiment to compare the growth rates of several strains of the fungus *Pythium*, ten replicate agar plates were inoculated with each strain. Immediately after inoculation two lines, crossing at right angles at the point of inoculation, were drawn on the base of each dish. At two-day intervals four radii were measured for each colony along the radiating lines and the mean radius for each colony calculated. The results for each strain are to be plotted to yield a growth curve and 95% confidence limits for the mean of each strain at each time of measurement are to be indicated by means of vertical lines through the corresponding points. The mean radius for each of the ten replicate colonies of Strain 'A' at eight days from inoculation were: 27, 24, 26, 28, 26, 25, 30, 28, 24, and 27 mm. With only ten replicates we compute ΣX and ΣX^2 directly from the measurements. (NB On many calculators ΣX and ΣX^2 may be accumulated simultaneously.)

$$N = 10; \quad \Sigma X = 265; \quad \text{and } \Sigma X^2 = 7055$$

$$\overline{X} = \Sigma X / N = 26.5 \text{ mm} \qquad s = \sqrt{\left(\dfrac{7055 - \dfrac{265^2}{10}}{9} \right)} = 1.9003$$

$$\text{S. E. of mean} = \dfrac{1.9003}{\sqrt{10}} = 0.601 \text{ mm}$$

95% confidence limits are $26.5 \pm t_{0.05} \times 0.601$ mm, where t has nine degrees of freedom.

i.e. $26.5 \pm 2.262 \times 0.601$

$\underline{26.5 \pm 1.36 \text{ mm}}$ (i.e. 25.14 to 27.86 mm)

Our best estimate of colony radius characteristic of Strain 'A' under the conditions of the experiment is 26.5 mm, and taking account of the variation between colonies and the number of replicates we estimate that there is a probability of 0.95 that the true mean lies within the range 25.14 mm to 27.86 mm.

NB The S. E. of the mean may be computed directly, thus:

S.E. of mean

$$= \sqrt{\left(\frac{\Sigma X^2 - \frac{(\Sigma X)^2}{N}}{N(N-1)} \right)} = \sqrt{\left(\frac{7055 - \frac{265^2}{10}}{10 \times 9} \right)} = 0.601 \text{ mm}$$

When plotting the sample mean we conventionally plot the confidence limits, thus:

```
      | ---- at 27.86
      x ---- at 26.50
      | ---- at 25.14
```

Much biological research is descriptive and although measurements are made and it is necessary to extrapolate from samples to populations no direct quantitative comparison between populations is called for. Such is often the case with the investigation of quantitative changes in the same system with time, e.g. growth of organisms, temporal changes in biological activity, etc. It is here that the attachment of confidence limits has its greatest value and a high proportion of the results published in graphical form have confidence limits plotted for each sample mean.

2.6   Probabilities of deviations

We sometimes need to estimate the probability of an individual observation, taken at random, or the mean of a random sample, deviating from a population mean by more than a certain amount. To do this we express the deviation in terms of standard deviation or standard error units (as appropriate) and treat the value obtained as d or where the standard deviation or standard error is estimated from a small sample as t. In computing confidence limits we multiply a standard deviation or standard error by the statistic (d or t) and obtain a deviation: here we divide a deviation by a standard deviation or standard error and equate the quotient to the statistic.

The oranges in a particular consignment are known to have a mean weight of 200 g and a standard deviation of 30 g. What is the probability of one fruit, taken at random, having a weight outside the range 150 to 250 g? Compute: $d = 50/30 = 1.667$, which corresponds approximately to the tabulated value (1.645) for $P = 0.1$. What is the probability of a random group of four fruit having a mean weight outside this range? The S.E. of the mean of four $= 30/\sqrt{4} = 15$; $d = 50/15 = 3.333$, which corresponds approximately to the tabulated value (3.291) for $P = 0.001$. These are both 'two-tailed' tests. If we are concerned only with the deviation in one direction we would need a 'one-tailed' test and would simply *halve* the tabulated probability value. Thus the probability of a single fruit *exceeding* 250 g is $0.1/2 = 0.05$.

We can frame our question in relation to the deviation of a sample mean from a fixed hypothetical value but obtain our estimate of the population variance from the sample itself, as in the following example. According to a particular hypothesis a certain ratio is *unity*. We make a series of independent replicate measurments of this ratio with the following results: 1.08, 0.95, 1.20, 1.01, 1.04, 1.13, 0.97, 1.09, 1.03, and 1.10. What is the probability that the mean of the random sample of ten measurements would deviate from the hypothetical mean by as much as or more than this particular one?

$\Sigma X = 10.6;\quad \overline{X} = 10.6/10 = 1.06$; deviation $= 1.06 - 1.00 = 0.06$
$\Sigma X^2 = 11.2874;\quad s = 0.07557$; S.E. of mean of 10 = 0.0239
$\therefore t = 0.06/0.0239 = 2.51$, corresponding to $P < 0.05$

The ratio is equated to **t** (rather than *d*) because *s* is estimated from a (small) sample. With an estimated probability of rather less then 0.05 we would reject (or at least seriously question) the hypothesis that the mean of the population of measurements *of which we have a sample* is unity. Note that by framing the question in relation to the observed deviation of the sample mean we have made this a test of significance.

Problems

2–1 An area of bog vegetation was surveyed and classified. A series of peat surface samples was taken and classified according to vegetation type. The peat samples were then analysed for a number of nutrient elements. The samples from Cotton Grass Bog gave the following values for total phosphate, in mg 100 g^{-1} dry weight.: 39.3, 46.6, 51.7, 46.0, 68.3, 58.0, 54.5, 62.4, 56.0, 48.2, 43.1, and 50.3. Compute the mean value and attach 95% confidence limits.

2–2 Chemical analyses of 25 replicate water samples provide an estimate of the mean concentration of Ca^{++} with 95% confidence limits of ± 2.0 mg 1^{-1}. How many more determinations are likely to be required for the 99% confidence limits to be of this magnitude?

2–3 A taxonomist wishes to estimate the mean length of a particular skull dimension for the animals in a population to within ± 1.0 mm with a probability of 0.95. He makes 36 measurements and computes the standard deviation to be 5.0 mm. What should he do then?

2–4 In a trial experiment a botanist determines the chlorophyll concentration in five replicate leaf discs. She decides that in further experiments the confidence limits should be approximately halved. By how much does she need to increase the number of replicates?

3 Continuous Distributions: Tests of Significance

3.1 Differences between the means of two large samples

Although the attachment of confidence limits suffices for some kinds of investigation (see § 2.5), more commonly comparisons between populations are called for and we need to apply tests of significance. It is important to understand clearly the nature of such tests. They have four essential features:

(i) An hypothesis, A, which leads to a particular expected result and an alternative one, B, which does not.

(ii) An observed result which deviates more or less from that expected from hypothesis A.

(iii) An estimate of the probability of obtaining a result which deviates from expectation as much as or more than the result actually observed.

(iv) A conclusion in the form of a choice between two alternatives. If the estimated probability, from (iii), is *low* (say $\leqslant 0.05$) the observed result is regarded as inconsistent with hypothesis A and it is rejected. The alternative hypothesis, B, is then adopted. If the estimated probability is *high* (say > 0.05) the observed result is regarded as consistent with hypothesis A and it is retained.

These four features may be identified in the example of section 1.4 and the last example of section 2.6.

In applying a test of significance to the difference between two sample means we employ the hypothesis that the two population means are equal (i.e. $\mu_1 = \mu_2$). It leads to the expectation that the sample means will be equal (i.e. $X_1 = X_2$) and deviations from this may be tested for significance. The alternative hypothesis of inequality leads to no exact expectation and cannot be tested directly. So, whatever the biological hypothesis, it is the hypothesis of no difference, sometimes called the 'null hypothesis', which is tested. The deviation of the result from expectation is simply $X_1 - X_2$. The estimate of probability must take into account the variability and numbers of individuals in both samples. Fortunately, if we have two normally-distributed populations the differences between two random individuals, one from one population and one from the other, are also normally-distributed. The standard deviation of that distribution (i.e. of the population of differences) is $\sigma_{1-2} = \sqrt{(\sigma_1^2 + \sigma_2^2)}$ which we can estimate as $s_{1-2} = \sqrt{(s_1^2 + s_2^2)}$. In comparing two means we require an estimate of the standard error of their difference. This is simply $\sqrt{(\sigma_1{}^2/N_1 + \sigma_2{}^2/N_2)}$ which we can estimate as $\sqrt{(s_1{}^2/N_1 + s_2{}^2/N_2)}$. This may be more easily understood as follows: σ^2, the square of the standard deviation, is called the *variance*. We have a simple rule that the variance of a sum *or* a difference is the sum of the separate variances. Thus, $\sigma_{1-2}{}^2 = \sigma_1{}^2 + \sigma_2{}^2$. Similarly, the variance of a mean is σ^2/N, so the variance of a difference between two means is $\sigma_1{}^2/N_1 + \sigma_2{}^2/N_2$ and the standard error of the difference is the square root of this.

In section 2.6 we tested the significance of the deviation of a sample mean from a fixed hypothetical value by computing

$$\frac{\text{deviation}}{\text{S.E. of sample mean}}$$

and equating this to t with $(N-1)$ degrees of freedom, where N was the number of measurements in the sample. The denominator is simply the S.E. of the sample mean because the fixed hypothetical value has no standard error. Had the sample been a large one (i.e. $N \geqslant 30$) we could have equated the quotient to the statistic d. When testing the significance of a difference between the means of two large samples we compute the corresponding quantity:

$$\frac{\text{difference between means}}{\text{S.E. of that difference}} = \frac{\overline{X}_1 - \overline{X}_2}{\sqrt{\left(\dfrac{s_1{}^2}{N_1} + \dfrac{s_2{}^2}{N_2}\right)}} \quad \text{and equate to } d$$

In Chapter 2 we examined data for the lengths of 100 bracken fronds (see § 2.1 and 2.4) from a certain area, Area 1. As part of the same investigation 80 fronds were measured from a second area, Area 2, with the following results: ΣX 80.8 and ΣX^2 83.60. We can compare the frond populations in the two areas, thus:

	Area 1	Area 2
ΣX	109.0	80.8
N	100	80
$\overline{X}$	1.09 m	1.01 m
ΣX^2	121.52	83.60

$$s^2 = \frac{121.52 - \dfrac{109^2}{100}}{99} = 0.0274 \qquad \frac{83.60 - \dfrac{80.8^2}{80}}{79} = 0.0252$$

$$d = \frac{1.090 - 1.010}{\sqrt{\left(\dfrac{0.0274}{100} + \dfrac{0.0252}{80}\right)}} = \frac{0.080}{0.0243} = \underline{3.292}$$

This value almost equals the tabulated value of d for $P = 0.001$ (3.291) so we conclude that there is a very highly significant difference between the mean frond lengths of the two populations. When the difference between the means has proved significant the S.E. of the difference may be used to attach confidence limits to the difference, thus S.E. of difference $= 0.024$. 95% confidence limits of the difference are $0.080 \pm 1.96 \times 0.024$ (0.033 to 0.127).

3.2   Differences between the means of two small samples – population variances assumed to be equal

It might be expected that when a comparison of the means of two small samples (i.e. when N_1 and $N_2 < 30$) was called for we could simply replace d in the test of the last section by t but this is not so. The use of t is fully valid only if we may assume the variances of the populations from which the samples were drawn are equal. We may often safely assume this to be the case, e.g. when we are dealing with rather small effects of different treatments on samples originally drawn from the same population. When we make the assumption of equal variance we make a combined estimate of it using the data from both samples, thus:

$$s_c^2 = \frac{[\Sigma X_1^2 - (\Sigma X_1)^2/N_1 + \Sigma X_2^2 - (\Sigma X_2)^2/N_2]}{N_1 + N_2 - 2} \equiv \frac{(\Sigma x_1^2 + \Sigma x_2^2)}{N_1 + N_2 - 2}$$

The estimated S.E. of the difference between sample means then becomes: $s_c \sqrt{(1/N_1 + 1/N_2)}$, and we thus compute:

$$t = \frac{\overline{X}_1 - \overline{X}_2}{s_c \sqrt{(1/N_1 + 1/N_2)}}, \text{ where } t \text{ has } (N_1 + N_2 - 2) \text{ degrees of freedom}$$

In section 2.5 we examined data for the radial growth of Strain A of *Pythium* after eight days. Unfortunately two plates of a Strain B became contaminated but the remaining eight plates gave the following results: ΣX 260 and ΣX^2 8481. We can compare the amount of growth of the two strains, thus:

	Strain A	Strain B
ΣX	265 mm	260 mm
N	10	8
$\overline{X}$	26.5 mm	32.5 mm
ΣX^2	7055	8481
Σx^2	$(7055 - 265^2/10) = 32.5$	$(8481 - 260^2/8) = 31.0$

$$s_c^2 = (32.5 + 31.0)/(10 + 8 - 2) = 3.969$$
$$s_c = \sqrt{3.969} = 1.99$$

$$t = \frac{26.5 - 32.5}{1.99 \sqrt{\left(\frac{1}{10} + \frac{1}{8}\right)}} = \frac{-6.0}{0.945} = -6.35, \text{ with 16 degrees of freedom}$$

This value is numerically greater than the tabulated value of t for $P = 0.001$ (4.015) so we conclude that there is a very highly significant difference between the amount of growth of the two strains.

95% confidence limits of the difference between the two strains are -6.0 mm $\pm t_{0.05} \times 0.945$, when t has 16 degrees of freedom. Thus: 95% confidence limits of difference are $-6.0 \pm 2.120 \times 0.945$ mm

i.e. $\underline{-6.0 \pm 2.00}$ (-4.0 to -8.0) mm

3.3 Differences between the means of two small samples – population variances *not* assumed to be equal

It frequently happens that we have reason to doubt the equality of the two population variances, either because the samples have been drawn from two independent populations, as in many surveys, or because the sample variances themselves are very different. (Such a difference may be tested for significance, § 9.4.) We may also expect inequality when the treatment effects are large or the data are not in the form of measurements but take the form of proportions, percentages or counts. In such cases the t-test as described in section 3.2 should *not* be used. There is no single, simple solution to this problem. Sometimes the answer lies in transformation of the data before analysis, section 9.4. More generally, a good approximate solution may be obtained by evaluating the expression used in section 3.1 and equating it to t with a reduced number of degrees of freedom, thus: we compute

$$\frac{\overline{X}_1 - \overline{X}_2}{\sqrt{(s_1^2/N_1 + s_2^2/N_2)}} = t, \text{ with } f \text{ degrees of freedom, where } f \text{ is given by:}$$

$1/f = u^2/(N_1 - 1) + (1 - u)^2/(N_2 - 1)$ and u by

$$u = \frac{s_1^2/N_1}{(s_1^2/N_1) + (s_2^2/N_2)}$$

Superficial examination of the limpets (*Patella vulgata*) on a rocky promontory suggested the hypothesis that the shells of animals on the exposed side tended to have a smaller maximum diameter than those on the sheltered side. A preliminary survey was carried out in which 15 limpets from the exposed side and 20 limpets from the sheltered side were compared. The results were as follows:

	Exposed	*Sheltered*
ΣX	744 mm	1024 mm
N	15	20
$\overline{X}$	49.6 mm	51.2 mm
ΣX^2	36 990	52 941
s^2	6.257	26.958

We note that the variance of the sample from the sheltered side (26.958) is greater than four times that of the sample from the exposed side (6.257) and as we have no *a priori* reason for supposing the population variances to be equal we employ the method described above.*

$$t = \frac{49.6 - 51.2}{\sqrt{[(6.257/15) + (26.958/20)]}} = \frac{-1.6}{1.3285} = -1.204$$

$$u = \frac{6.257/15}{(6.257/15) + (26.958/20)} = 0.2363$$

$$1/f = (0.2363^2/14) + (1 - 0.2363)^2/19) = 0.0347$$
$$f = 28.83, \text{ or to the nearest integer } \underline{29}$$

The computed value of *t* is less than the tabulated value for $P = 0.1$ and 29 degrees of freedom, so we conclude that the difference of 1.6 mm between the sample means is non-significant. It is possible that, with larger numbers of replicates and greater care taken to collect animals from one level on the shore, a significant result might be obtained.

3.4   Confidence limits in the comparison of treatment means

In the same way that confidence limits are not absolute ranges but relate only to selected probability levels, so tests of significance do not always lead to correct conclusions. In using 95% confidence limits one must accept that *on average* the true mean will lie *outside* the limits once in every twenty tests. Similarly, when employing tests of significance one must accept the real possibility (and the long-term inevitability) of error. Such errors are of two kinds:

(i) erroneous rejection of the null hypothesis, i.e. reaching the conclusion that the population means are different when they are, in fact, equal: *Type 1 error*.

(ii) erroneous retention of the null hypothesis, i.e. reaching the conclusion that the population means are equal when, in fact, they are not: *Type 2 error*.

In making a test of significance the probabilities of making Type 1 and

* Applying the test of section 9.4 $26.958/6.257 = 4.31 > 3.66$ the tabulated value of F with 15 14 degrees of freedom and $P = 0.01$ so difference significant at $P < 0.02$.

Type 2 errors are affected by the critical probability selected, e.g. to select $P = 0.01$ in place of $P = 0.05$ decreases the probability of making a Type 1 error but increases the probability of making a Type 2 error. Ideally, selection of probability level should be made on consideration of the relative costs of making the two sorts of error.

Some biologists tend to make comparisons between sample means by examination of confidence limits. If the confidence limits of the two means do not meet, Fig. 3–1a, the difference between the two means is considered to be significant. If the confidence limits overlap, Fig. 3–1b, the difference is considered to be non significant.

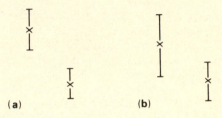

(a)   (b)

Fig. 3–1   Confidence limits plotted for two pairs of means: (a) not meeting, (b) overlapping.

The implication is that these tests are made at the probability level used in attaching the confidence limits. This is not correct as the following example illustrates:

	Sample 1	Sample 2
ΣX	160.000	228.192
N	16	16
$\overline{X}$	10.000	14.262
ΣX^2	1840.000	3494.474
s	4.000	4.000
S. E. of mean	$4/\sqrt{16} = 1.000$	$4/\sqrt{16} = 1.000$
95% confidence limits	$10.000 \pm 2.131 \times 1.000$ i.e. 12.131 to 7.869	$14.262 \pm 2.131 \times 1.000$ i.e. 16.393 to 12.131

Where 2.131 is the tabulated value of t for 15 degrees of freedom. Note that the 95% confidence limits just meet, at 12.131. Now apply the t-test:

$$s_c^2 = \frac{1}{16 + 16 - 2} \left(1840.000 - \frac{160^2}{16} + 3494.474 - \frac{228.192^2}{16} \right)$$
$$= 16$$
$$\therefore s_c = 4 \text{ (as would be expected).}$$
$$t = \frac{10.000 - 14.262}{4\sqrt{1/16 + 1/16}} = \frac{-4.262}{1.414} = \underline{-3.014} \quad \begin{array}{l} \text{with 30 degrees} \\ \text{of freedom.} \\ \text{giving } P < 0.01 \end{array}$$

The effective probability level of the test is thus greatly lowered, but by an amount which is generally unknown. The probablity of making a Type 2 error is increased by an unknown amount. The difference arises because of the non-linear distribution of probability between the confidence limits and, to a lesser extent, to the difference in the number of degrees of freedom. Clearly the practice is undesirable. When a comparison is needed it should be made by means of the appropriate test of significance.

3.5   Paired-sample test

We have considered several forms of test applicable to comparisons between two sample means. In all of them we have had two independent samples and have computed the ratio of the difference between the sample means to the estimated standard error of that difference. The sensitivity of such a test depends on the number of replicates and the level of variation between them. Some investigations lend themselves to an experimental design in which the replicates, one from each population, are paired. This can greatly decrease the effect of variation. If we wished to compare the effects of two different diets on the live weight gains of calves we might experience difficulty in obtaining the necessary population of calves of the same breed and age from which to draw two random samples. To use a paired design we would need a number of calf twins. We would feed one calf in each pair on the first diet and the other on the second. Because we are concerned only with the *differences* in weight gain between the pairs of twins we are free to include in the experiment twins of different breed and rather different age. The null hypothesis tested is that the *mean difference* between the pairs is zero. We compute:

$$\frac{\text{mean difference}}{\text{S.E. of mean difference}} = \frac{\bar{Z}}{s_Z / \sqrt{N}} = t, \text{ with } (N-1) \text{ degrees of freedom}$$

where Z is the difference between the individuals of a pair, and N is the number of pairs. When computing Z as $\Sigma Z / N$ account must be taken of the sign of Z.

The advantage of the paired test depends on the pairing of individuals that are more similar to one another than to the other individuals receiving the same treatment. In some investigations the same biological individual can constitute a pair by being tested both before and after treatment. The following example illustrates such a test. In an investigation on the effect of eating on pulse rate a student measured the pulse rate of a group of people, ranging from young children to elderly adults, both before and after they had eaten a substantial meal. The following results were obtained, in beats min^{-1}.

Subject	1	2	3	4	5	6	7	8	9	10	11	12	13	14
Before	105	79	79	103	87	74	73	82	78	86	77	76	79	104
After	109	87	86	109	100	82	80	90	90	93	81	81	90	110
Diff (Z)	+4	+8	+7	+6	+13	+8	+7	+8	+12	+7	+4	+5	+11	+6

$$N = 14; \quad \Sigma Z = +106; \quad \overline{Z} = +7.571; \quad \Sigma Z^2 = 902$$

$$s_Z = \sqrt{\left(\frac{902 - 106^2/14}{13}\right)} = \underline{2.766}$$

$$t = \frac{+7.571}{2.766/\sqrt{14}} = \underline{10.24},$$ which greatly exceeds the tabulated value of t for 13 degrees of freedom and $P = 0.001$

We conclude that the observed *mean increase* in pulse rate after food is very highly significant. (See also Problem 3–3.)

Problems

3–1 Re-analyse the data of the example in section 3.1 by means of a t-test

3–2 It was suspected that the stoats (*Mustela erminea*) on two neighbouring islands were of different races. A number of animals were trapped and some body measurements made. The tail lengths, in mm, are given below.

Island J:	101, 111, 105, 121, 107, 99, 103, 117, 123, 100, 109, 96, 106, 98, 115
Island K:	101, 106, 107, 96, 97, 100, 103, 100, 101, 95, 102, 104, 109, 93, 99, 102, 101, 99, 96, 98

Compare the two sample means without assuming the population variances to be equal.

3–3 Re-analyse the data of the example in section 3.4, taking no account of the pairing, i.e. by a normal t-test. How does the result compare with that of the paired-sample test?

3–4 In studies on moor matgrass (*Nardus stricta*) it was suspected that the grass, which grew in well-defined colonies, grew where the soil was *locally deeper*. To test this two soil depth measurements were made for each of 50 colonies, one within the colony and one just outside. The sum of the differences for the 50 pairs of measurements, ΣZ, was $+637$ cm. The sum of the squares of the differences, ΣZ^2, was 14 433. Examine the significance of the mean difference by means of the paired-sample test.

4 Discontinuous Distributions: Binomial Distribution

4.1 When do we meet this distribution?

There are many occasions in biology on which we distinguish two mutually-exclusive categories, e.g. present $v.$ absent; alive $v.$ dead; germinated or hatched $v.$ dormant; pigmented $v.$ unpigmented, etc. When we examine a group of such individuals and count the numbers falling into their two categories we can expect to obtain data that tend to be binomially distributed. We have met two examples already in Chapter 1: one involving beetles that moved either to high humidity or to low (see § 1.3) and the other involving children that were either male or female (Problem 1–2). It is common practice to convert the observed frequencies into proportions and percentages, e.g. percentage mortality.

4.2 Standard error

Having made observations on limited samples we need, as with measurement data, to make statements and draw conclusions about populations. With measurement data, having made the assumption that the probability distribution of the population was at least approximately normal, we used the information from the sample to calculate $\bar{X}$ (sample mean) as an estimate of μ (population mean) and s (sample standard deviation) as an estimate of σ (population standard deviation) which together defined the particular normal distribution. By treating deviations as multiples of s we were able to use tabulated information about the probability distribution common to all normally-distributed variables. This information (in the form of tables of d and t) then enabled us to attach confidence limits and make tests of significance.

We have already seen (section 1.3) that a binomial probability distribution can be defined by expanding an expression of the form $(p + q)^n$, where p is the probability of a single individual, taken at random, falling into one category—conventionally distinguished as a *success*, $q = 1 - p$, the probability of it falling into the other—conventionally regarded as a *failure*, and n is the number of individuals in the group. The probability distribution is thus completely defined by n and p. There are several ways of using this information to attach confidence limits and to make tests of significance.

A binomial probability distribution describes the relative probabilities of different numbers of successes (from n to 0) when the probability of any one individual scoring a success is p (Fig. 1–1). It is clear that the mean number of successes is pn and it may be shown that the standard deviation of the number of successes (or failures) in a group is $\sqrt{(pqn)}$. As n is determined by the investigator and p (and q) can be estimated from observation of a single group it is possible to make confidence statements from the evidence of one group only. If, in a germination test, we set a sample of 400 seeds and 320 germinate the estimated percentage germination of the population from which the sample was drawn would be $(320/400) \times 100 = 80\%$. We could estimate p empirically (see § 1.2) as $320/400 = 0.8$, and $q = 0.2$. The estimated standard deviation of the observed number germinating is thus $\sqrt{(0.8 \times 0.2 \times 400)} = 8.0$. But this is the S.D. of the number germinating out of 400 so the S.D., or S.E.* of the percentage germination is $8 \times 100/400 = 2.0$. There is another and more rapid way of achieving the same result. Each group observed can yield its own estimate of p, and it can be shown that the S.D. of these estimates is $\sqrt{(pq/n)}$. As the percentage germination is simply $100p$ the estimated S.E. of the percentage germination is simply $100 \sqrt{(pq/n)}$, or $\sqrt{(PQ/n)}$ where P and Q are p and q expressed as percentages.

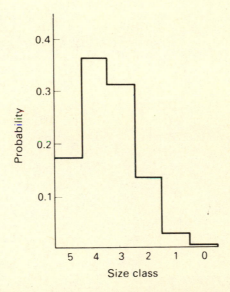

Fig. 4–1 Probability distribution for $(p + q)^n$, where $p = 0.7$ *and* $n = 5$.

* A standard error is only the standard deviation of a quantity in which we are interested.

4.3   Confidence limits

When attaching confidence limits to a sample mean of normally-distributed measurements we multiplied the standard error of the mean by tabulated values of d or t so as to define the range within which we predicted 95°/o or 99°/o of values would lie. The binomial distribution of probability is discontinuous and generally not symmetrical. See Fig. 4–1 which illustrates the distribution for $(0.7 + 0.3)^5$. However, when seeking to attach confidence limits to our estimate of percentage germination in the example in section 4.2 we would need the probability distribution corresponding to $(0.8 + 0.2)^{400}$. The outline of the histogram for this expansion would be an almost symmetrical nearly smooth curve and would approximate closely a normal curve with $\mu = 320$ and $\sigma = 8$. In fact, it may be shown that a binomial distribution tends to normality as n increases, provided that neither p nor q approaches 0 or 1. In practice, provided that neither pn nor qn is less than 50, we may use the value of d to attach confidence limits. See also Fig. 4–2 which illustrates the probability distribution for the expansion $(0.6 + 0.4)^{60}$, giving $pn = 36$ and $qn = 24$.

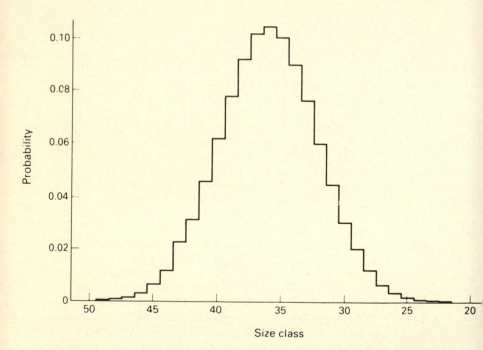

Fig. 4 2   Probability distribution for $(p + q)^n$ when $p = 0.6$ *and* $n = 60$, *so* $pn = 36$ *and* $qn = 24$.

So, approximate 95% confidence limits of the percentage germination in the example in section 4.2 are $80\% \pm 1.96 \times 2.0$, i.e. $80\% \pm 3.92$ or from 76.08 to 83.92%. A rather better approximation may be obtained thus:

$$\text{Confidence limits of } p \text{ are } \quad \frac{p + \dfrac{a^2}{2n} \pm \dfrac{a}{\sqrt{n}} \sqrt{(pq + a^2/4n)}}{1 + a^2/n}$$

where n = number of observations in group

and a = tabulated value of d for chosen probability,
          e.g. 1.96 for 95% and 2.576 for 99% limits.

For $n = 400$, $p = 0.8$ and $a = 1.96$ this yields 95% limits of p of from 0.758 to 0.836, and hence 95% limits for percentage germination of from 75.8 to 83.6%.

(NB For smaller samples and/or where p approaches 0 or 1 confidence limits may be read from Table 1.4.1 of SNEDECOR and COCHRAN (1967), Table IX of SOKAL and ROHLF (1973), or Table W of ROHLF and SOKAL (1969).)

4.4   Tests of hypothesis

In many investigations when we observe the frequencies with which the n individuals of a group fall into two categories we do so with the object of testing an hypothesis. Frequently this is a null hypothesis, i.e. $p = q = 0.5$ (see § 1.4) There are several ways of testing deviations from expectation for significance.

One, sometimes called the 'exact method', takes the form of computing the probability of the observed result and others deviating equally or more from expectation. The individual probabilities are computed as terms of the binomial expansion $(p + q)^n$, where p is the *hypothetical* probability of a success. The general formula for a term of expansion is:

$$\frac{n!}{k!(n-k)!} \, p^k \, q^{(n-k)}$$

where k is the particular number of successes and ! denotes 'factorial'. If the direction of any deviation can be predicted a 'one-tailed' test is called for and only the extreme terms in the direction of the observed deviation summed. Otherwise a 'two-tailed' test is called for and the two groups of extreme terms are computed and summed (see § 1.4 and Problem 1–2).

A second method employs a normal approximation. Suppose that out of a total of n observations we record X successes when our hypothesis leads us to expect pn. We could estimate the S.E. of X as $\sqrt{(pqn)}$, compute the ratio (deviation)/(S.E. of deviation) and equate to d. As with the use of d in computing confidence limits this would involve approximation. This can be improved by applying a correction for continuity which takes the form of reducing the magnitude of the deviation by 0.5. So we compute: $d = (|X - pn| - 0.5)/\sqrt{(pqn)}$ where $|\quad|$ denotes the *positive* difference between the enclosed values. When $p = q = 0.5$ this reduces to: $d = (|X - (n - X)| - 1.0)/\sqrt{n}$. (A third method, employing the statistic χ^2, will be described in § 6.2.)

4.5   Differences between proportions and percentages

As with the normal distribution itself in which a method for testing the significance of a deviation from a hypothetical value (see § 2.6) was extended to a test of significance between two sample means (see § 3.1), so the method involving normal approximation, above, can be developed to examine differences between proportions and percentages. The resulting method will not be included here because it is applicable to large samples only and is less convenient than one, using χ^2, that compares directly the observed and expected frequencies, and is described in section 7.2.

4.6   Problems and possibilities

We have seen that provided certain assumptions are made we can attach confidence limits and carry out tests of significance on the evidence of a single (large) sample. It sometimes happens however that we have data for a number of replicate (small) samples and are not sure what assumptions may be safely made about them. If we can satisfy ourselves that our samples are unbiassed and that the events observed were *independent of one another* (i.e. the occurrence of one success did not make another either more or less likely) then we may sum the data for the replicate samples and treat the whole as a single large sample using the methods in sections 4.2, 4.3, and 4.4. If we are not satisfied there are two courses open to us:

(i) The data for a series of individual samples may be treated in the same way as measurements on a continuous scale and analysed by the methods of Chapters 2 and 3. Transformation of the data, e.g. to $\sin^{-1}\sqrt{p}$, may be called for, especially when the recorded frequencies are low. The matter is dealt with in section 9.4.

(ii) The data for a series of individual samples may be used to *test the hypothesis of independence*. If we carry out of a series of N trials, recording the number of successes X out of a total of n at each trial, on the hypothesis of independence we would expect the frequencies of the different numbers of successes to approach the terms of the expansion $N(p + q)^n$, where $p = \Sigma X/Nn$. Having made our N trials we are in a position to compare the observed and expected frequencies. The *goodness-of-fit* test for this will be described in Chapter 6. More simply, and using a test that is already familiar to us we can compare the *observed variance* of the number of successes per trial (s_X^2, estimated as $(\Sigma X^2 - (\Sigma X^2/N)/(N-1)$ (i.e. $\Sigma x^2/(N-1)$) with the *expected variance* if their distribution is binomial, i.e. pqn. We may test the significance of the difference between the observed and expected variances in the usual way, i.e. (difference)/(S.E. of difference) $= t$, with $(N-1)$ degrees of freedom. The S.E. of the difference may be computed directly from pqn and N, and is:

$$\sqrt{\left(\frac{2(pqn)^2}{N-1} + \frac{pqn(1-6pq)}{N}\right)}$$

Even more conveniently, especially when N is not too large, we may compute $(\Sigma X^2 - (\Sigma X)^2/N)/pqn$, (i.e. $\Sigma x^2/pqn$) and equate it to χ^2 with $(N-1)$ degrees of freedom. (See Problems 4–7 and 4–8.)

The fact that a binomial distribution is entirely determined by p and n opens up useful possibilities of estimation. We have seen already (§ 1.4 and 4.4) that all terms of an expansion may be computed from a hypothetical value of p. The same may be done from an observed (estimated) value of p, or p itself may be estimated from hypothetical or observed values of individual terms. (See Problems 4–5. and 4–6.)

Problems

4–1   30 cysts of *Cotylurus erraticus* (a fish parasite) out of 50 were found to hatch under a particular set of experimental conditions. Calculate the percentage hatchability and attach 95% confidence limits to your estimate using *both* methods in section 4.3.

4–2   The cover of daisies (*Bellis perennis*) in a lawn was estimated by recording 'hits' or 'misses' for 200 randomly located pins (= point-quadrats), and 50 'hits' were recorded. Compute the estimated percentage cover for the lawn and attach 95% confidence limits to your estimate using *both* methods in section 4.3. How many point-quadrats would have to be examined for the 95% confidence limits to lie within 2% of one another (i.e. $\pm\ 1.0\%$)?

4–3   100 seeds were taken from a large consignment and tested for germination. They all germinated. What can be said about the germinability of the rest of the seeds in the consignment? (Try attaching confidence limits to the percentage germination.)

4–4   The behaviour of 20 male insects was examined in a choice experiment, in which a volatile chemical X which could possibly act as a sex attractant was presented in one of the two arms of the chamber. 15 insects moved towards X. Carry out tests of significance, treating them as 'two-tailed' because X might prove to be a repellant. Use *both* tests in section 4.4.

4–5 A wholesale seed merchant received a complaint from a retailer about some annual flower seeds sold enclosed in paper strips ready for planting, each containing ten seeds. The retailer reported that in only 50"₀ of the strips did all the seeds germinate. Assuming this report to be accurate estimate the percentage germination of the seed batch used in preparation of the strips.

4–6 In a certain multiple-choice examination each question has listed five answers of which one and only one is correct. There are six questions all of equal weight and 50"₀ is required for passing. Compute the probability of a student passing the examination if he answers each question at random.

4–7 Seeds were taken from ripe tomatoes and set to germinate, still surrounded by their gelatinous placental tissue, on moistened filter paper. 400 seeds were set singly and 344 germinated after twelve days. 400 seeds were also set as 200 isolated pairs, with the following result, after twelve days:

Number germinated in pair:	2	1	0
Number of pairs:	82	76	42

Compute the percentage germination for both treatments. How would you test the significance of the difference between them? Test the hypothesis that the seeds in pairs behaved independently of one another, using the methods in section 4.6. (The goodness-of-fit to the expected binomial frequencies will be tested in Problem 6–3.)

4–8 In the course of an investigation of the effect of management on the establishment and spread of white clover (*Trifolium repens*) in grass-clover lays the percentage cover of clover was estimated in a certain experimental plot. To reduce the physical labour of locating, observing and recording the large number of point-quadrats a linear group of five point-quadrats was used with points 10 cm apart. This was located randomly 200 times and the number of 'hits' by each point-quadrat group recorded, with the following results:

Number of 'hits':	5	4	3	2	1	0
Frequency:	4	13	26	48	74	35

Compute the estimated percentage cover of clover for the plot. How would you attach confidence limits to the estimate? Test the hypothesis of 'independence' using the methods in section 4.6. Suggest an explanation of your result in terms of the distribution pattern of the clover. (The goodness-of-fit to the expected binomial frequencies will be tested in Problem 6–4.)

5 Discontinuous Distributions: Poisson Distribution

5.1 When do we meet this distribution?

When we count blood cells or microorganisms within a square of a haemocytometer slide or when we count emissions of a radioactive sample within a certain time we are counting randomly-distributed items or events in an unbiassed sample. Such counts have a particular kind of discontinuous distribution in which the probabilities of obtaining a count of a certain size (from 0 upwards) is given by the corresponding term of the Poisson expansion: $e^{-m}(1, m, m^2/2!, m^3/3!, m^4/4!$. etc.), where m is the mean number of items or events.

5.2 Standard error

We have seen how a normal distribution may be defined in terms of its mean and standard deviation, and a binomial distribution in terms of its mean (pn) and number in a group (n). The Poisson distribution is peculiar in that it is completely defined by one parameter, its mean. Not only this, the variance of the counts is equal to their mean, i.e. $\sigma^2 = \mu$. In practice we can make a single count, say X, and use it to estimate both μ and σ^2. The S.E. of X as an estimate of μ, is then estimated as $\sqrt{X}$.

5.3 Confidence limits

Like the binomial distribution the Poisson distribution is discontinuous but always to some degree asymmetrical. These features are most marked when m is low, see Fig. 5–1. As m increases so the distribution becomes more nearly symmetrical and, like the binomial, approaches a normal distribution. So, provided that the number counted is large ($\geqslant 50$, say) confidence limits may be attached using d, thus: 95% limits of μ are $X \pm 1.96\sqrt{X}$. So if 150 emissions are counted for a radioactive sample in one minute we may estimate μ as $X = 150$, estimate the S.E. of the number of counts per minute as $\sqrt{X} = \sqrt{150} = 12.25$, and the 95% limits of μ as $150 \pm 1.96 \times 12.25$, i.e. 150 ± 24, or 126 to 174 counts per minute. See also Fig. 5–2.

As with the binomial distribution an improved estimate is possible, this time with very little additional computation. Confidence limits of μ are $X + a^2/2 \pm a\sqrt{(X + a^2/4)}$, where a is the value of d for the chosen

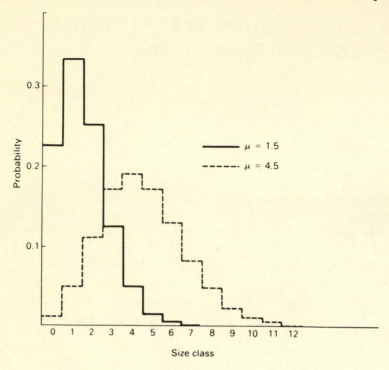

Fig. 5-1 Poisson distribution for $\mu = 1.5$ and $\mu = 4.5$.

probability, e.g. 1.96 for 95% limits. For the above example the 95% limits are:

$$150 + 1.96^2/2 \pm 1.96 \sqrt{(150 + 1.96^2/4)} = 127.84 \text{ to } 176.00 \text{ counts min}^{-1}.$$

5.4 Test of hypothesis

The need to test agreement of a count with hypothesis does not arise very often but if needed we can again compute the ratio of the deviation to its estimated standard error. Approximation is again improved by a correction for continuity, thus: $d = (|X - \mu| - 0.5)/\sqrt{\mu}$, where X is the observed count and μ the hypothetical mean count. (See Problem 5-3.)

5.5 Comparison of two Poisson counts

For a test of significance between two Poisson counts in samples of equal size we may compute:

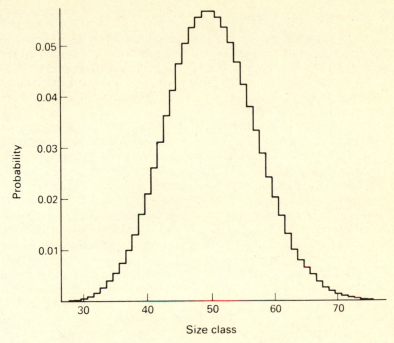

Fig. 5–2 Poisson distribution for $\mu = 50$.

$$d = \frac{|X_1 - (X_1 + X_2)/2| - 0.5}{\sqrt{[(X_1 + X_2)/4]}},$$

where X_1 and X_2 are the two counts. If the samples are unequal, and of sizes Y_1 and Y_2, we compute:

$$d = \frac{|X_1 - (X_1 + X_2)(Y_1/(Y_1 + Y_2)| - 0.5}{\sqrt{[(X_1 + X_2)(Y_1/(Y_1 + Y_2))(Y_2/(Y_1 + Y_2))]}}$$

To compare single sample counts of two *Chlorella* suspensions, of 50 and 30, the samples being of the same volume, we compute:

$$d = \frac{|50 - (50 + 30)/2| - 0.5}{\sqrt{[(50 + 30)/4]}} = \underline{2.124}, \text{ giving } P < 0.05$$

We conclude that the densities of the two *Chlorella* suspensions were different. (See also Problem 5–2.)

5.6   Problems and possibilities

If we have counts for a series of replicate samples, provided that we can satisfy ourselves that the samples are equal and unbiassed, and that the items or events counted were randomly distributed, we may sum the data for the replicate samples and treat the whole as a single large sample, employing the methods in section 5.2 to 5.5. If we are not satisfied there are two courses open to us:

(i) Treat the data for the series of samples in the same way as measurements on a continuous scale, using the methods of Chapters 2 and 3. Transformation of the data, to $\sqrt{X}$ or $\sqrt{(X+0.5)}$, before analysis may be called for. This matter is dealt with in section 9.4.

(ii) The data for a series of individual samples may be used to *test* the hypothesis subject to doubt, e.g. randomness. If we sample a population of plants by means of a series of equal area samples (quadrats) and count the numbers of individuals in each we can test the hypothesis that the plants are randomly distributed. If they are not we can with reason go on to investigate why they are not. We may compare the observed frequencies with which the different counts (0's, 1's, 2's, 3's and etc.) are made against the frequencies which would be expected if the population were randomly distributed. These are given by the expansion: $N e^{-m}(1, m, m^2/2!, m^3/3!$, and etc.), where m is the mean number of plants observed per sample and N is the number of samples. Alternatively we may compute the ratio of the observed variance of the counts, estimated as $(\Sigma X^2 - (\Sigma X)^2/N)/(N-1)$ (i.e. $\Sigma x^2/(N-1)$) and the expected variance estimated as $m = \bar{X} = \Sigma X/N$ and compare this with the expected ratio of unity for a Poisson distribution ($\sigma^2/\mu = 1.0$). Deviations from unity may be tested in the usual way, i.e. $[(\text{variance/mean})-1]/\text{S.E.}$ of difference $= t$, with $(N-1)$ degrees of freedom. The S.E. of the variance/mean ratio depends entirely on N and is $\sqrt{[2/(N-1)]}$. More conveniently we may compute $\Sigma x^2/\bar{X}$ and equate to χ^2 with $(N-1)$ degrees of freedom. (See Problem 5–4.)

As a Poisson distribution is determined by its mean alone it is often possible to make useful estimates from very limited evidence. It is possible to estimate μ from the frequency of counts of one size, e.g. the number of 0's. Conversely, given the value of μ estimates may be made of the frequencies in one or a selected group of size classes. In one method of estimating mutation rate in bacteria mutation is indicated by the multiplication of the organism rendering its liquid medium turbid. It is possible only to distinguish between no mutation and one or more mutations because turbidity in any one tube may be due to 1, 2, 3, or more mutations. Tubes of liquid medium are inoculated with equal numbers of bacteria (equal samples). Mutations occur randomly (random distribution) so we assume the frequency distribution of mutants in the tubes to approach a Poisson distribution. The number of tubes which remain clear, i.e. in which no mutations occur, is equated to Ne^{-m}, where N is the total number of tubes. We can compute m, the mean number of mutations per tube, and knowing the number of bacteria used in inoculation, the mutation rate. It is necessary, of course, to adjust the number of bacteria per tube so that the mean number of mutations per tube is low. (See also Problem 5–5.)

Problems

5–1 In planning to study seasonal fluctuation in density of the several most important plankton organisms in a pond, a student considered that for each organism 95% confidence limits of approximately $\pm 5\%$ would be required. How many organisms of each species should be counted per water sample? (Assume random distribution of organisms.)

5–2 A radioactive sample Y was counted for five minutes and 165 emissions were recorded. Another sample Z was counted for only three minutes and 120 emissions were recorded. Compute and compare the emission rates. Are they significantly different at $P < 0.05$?

5–3 It is known from repeated checks over a long time period that the mean background count rate of a particular piece of radioactive counting equipment is 285 per hour. A user suspects that the equipment has been contaminated, makes a background count for one hour and records 317. Does this significantly exceed the long-term mean?

5–4 During an autecological study of a particular plant species, counts were made of the numbers of individuals present in 200 random area samples. Results:

No. of plants	0	1	2	3	4	5	6	7	8	9	10
Frequency	31	48	44	33	18	13	7	3	2	1	0

Compute the estimated plant density as the mean number of plants per sample. How would you attach confidence limits to the estimate? Test the hypothesis of randomness using the methods in section 5.6. (The goodness-of-fit to the expected Poisson distribution will be tested in Problem 6.5.)

5–5 It is known that on average there are 1.5 weed seeds per packet of a certain lot of vegetable seeds. What is the probability of a packet containing more than three weed seeds?

6 Analysis of Frequencies: Single Classification

6.1 Two frequencies and more

The data resulting from biological surveys and experiments are of two main types. In one, each individual, item or event is characterized by a measurement or some other kind of quantitative assessment. In the other type, each individual is placed into a particular class and interest is centred on the frequencies with which individuals fall into these. We have learnt, in Chapters 2 and 3, how to deal with measurement data for one or two samples. In Chapters 4 and 5 we have seen how these methods may be extended to cover situations in which the assessment of a sample (and hence of its parent population) is made in terms of counts of individuals in certain classes, e.g. percentage germination. In many biological investigations however the hypotheses we have to test have nothing to do with quantitative assessment of individuals or samples but relate directly to the probabilities, and hence the frequencies, with which individuals or observations fall into specified classes.

Essentially we have a finite number of observations which are classified into two or more classes. Hypothesis leads us to expect the observations to fall into these classes in particular proportions, and hence in particular frequencies. In general there are deviations between the observed and expected frequencies so we need both an overall measure of the deviations and a method of estimating the probability of such deviations from expectation occuring in order to provide a test of significance. A solution was proposed by Karl Pearson in 1899 in the form of the χ^2 (Chi^2) statistic. Overall measures of deviation between observed and expected frequencies are computed in several different ways and the resulting values equated to χ^2 for which critical values are tabulated. The derivation of χ^2 is complex so we shall concern ourselves primarily with its uses and hope that its relationship with the other statistics will gradually become clear.

6.2 Goodness-of-fit: two classes

The simplest kind of situation is that in which a set of observations is classified into two (mutually-exclusive) classes. We have to compare the two observed frequencies with the two frequencies expected by hypothesis. We can compute $\Sigma[(O-E)^2/E]$ and equate this to χ^2 with one degree of freedom, where O is the observed frequency and E the corresponding expected frequency.

Gregor Mendel raised 929 plants resulting from the self-fertilization of pea plants heterozygous for flower colour: 705 of these had coloured flowers and the remaining 224 had white flowers. Are these numbers of offspring consistent with the hypothesis of a 3:1 ratio of coloured to white?

Class	Observed frequency	Expected frequency	Deviation
Coloured	705	696.75	+8.25
White	224	232.25	−8.25
(Total)	(929)	(929.00)	(0.00)

$$\chi^2 = \frac{(+8.25)^2}{696.75} + \frac{(-8.25)^2}{232.25} = 0.3907, \text{ with one degree of freedom,}$$
$$\text{giving } P > 0.5$$

This leads to the conclusion that the deviations from expectation are not significant and therefore that the observed results are consistent with the original hypothesis.

The χ^2 distribution, like the normal distribution, is continuous whereas the distribution of the computed values, being based on frequencies, is discontinuous. There is a resulting tendency to under estimate probabilities and thus increase the liklihood of Type 1 errors (see § 3.4). This tendency can be corrected by applying the correction for continuity, which takes the form of reducing the magnitude of all deviations by 0.5 before squaring. Applied to the above example this becomes:

$$\chi^2 = \frac{(8.25 - 0.5)^2}{696.75} + \frac{(8.25 - 0.5)^2}{232.25} = 0.3448, \text{ with one degree of}$$
$$\text{freedom, giving } P > 0.5$$

In this example the conclusion is unaffected by the application of the correction.

With only two classes the test in section 4.4 is applicable, thus:

$$d = \frac{8.25 - 0.5}{\sqrt{(0.25 \times 0.75 \times 929)}} = \frac{7.75}{13.20} = 0.5872, \text{ giving } P > 0.5.$$

In this test we computed (deviation)/(S.E. of deviation) and equated to d. We could also compute (deviation)^2/(variance of deviation) and equate to

χ^2 with one degree of freedom, thus: (including correction) $\chi^2 = (8.25 - 0.5)^2/(0.25 \times 0.75 \times 929) = 0.3448$, giving $P > 0.5$. Note that d (0.5872) is equal to $\sqrt{\chi^2}$ ($\sqrt{0.3448}$) with one degree of freedom. We have already met χ^2 in the form of $\Sigma(\text{deviation})^2/(\text{variance})$ in sections 4.6 and 5.6.

6.3   Goodness-of-fit: more than two classes

With more than two classes the necessary additional terms are included in the χ^2 sum and there are additional degrees of freedom for the test. The correction for continuity is not applied in tests with more than one degree of freedom.

Mendel reported the following results for the dihybrid cross with peas: *round/yellow* 315, *round/green* 108, *wrinkled/yellow* 101 and *wrinkled/green* 32. Are these results consistent with the hypothesis of independent segregation and the simple dominance of *yellow* over *green* and *round* over *wrinkled*?, i.e. are they consistent with the ratios 9 : 3 : 3 : 1?

Class	Observed frequency	Expected frequency	Deviation
Round/yellow	315	312.75	+2.25
Round/green	108	104.25	+3.75
Wrinkled/yellow	101	104.25	−3.25
Wrinkled/green	32	34.75	−2.75
(Total)	(556)	(556.00)	(0.00)

$$\chi^2 = \frac{2.25^2}{312.75} + \frac{3.75^2}{104.25} + \frac{(-3.25)^2}{104.25} + \frac{(-2.75)^2}{34.75} = \underline{0.470}$$

with three degrees of freedom, giving $P > 0.9$

This means that even if the hypothesis is true deviations of this magnitude or greater would be expected to occur in repeated trials more often than 9 times out of 10. That such close agreement between observed and expected frequencies should occur from time to time is to be expected but if such very high probabilities are met with repeatedly bias in recording should be looked for.

6.4   Lower limit of expected frequencies

The use of χ^2 involves an approximation in that it is based on the assumption that the distribution of the expected frequencies is normal. This approximation clearly does not hold if expected frequencies are small. Conventionally a lower limit of five has been used (but see § 7.3.) If one or more of the expected frequencies fall below five the smaller groups are pooled until this condition is fulfilled, the sum of the several expected frequencies being compared with the sum of the corresponding observed frequencies. In combining classes in this way degrees of freedom are lost, the number of degrees of freedom being based on the number of comparisons made. (See Problems 6–4 and 6–5.)

6.5   Expected frequencies derived from observations

When the expected frequencies are determined only by the total number of observations and the hypothesis the number of degrees of freedom available for the test is *one less* than the number of comparisons made (see § 6.2 and 6.3). It frequently happens however that the expected frequencies depend on an unknown parameter which has to be estimated from the data, the goodness-of-fit of which is being tested. We have already met two such cases: one in section 5.6 where the mean of a Poisson distribution was estimated and the other in section 4.6 which involved the estimation of p in a binomial distribution. The effect of estimating a parameter in this way is to reduce by one the number of degrees of freedom for the test. In such cases the number of degrees of freedom is *two less* than the number of comparisons made. (See Problems 6–3, 6–4 and 6–5.)

This may be understood by considering a putative binomial distribution of group size n, the p value of which is subject to a hypothesis. Given the number of successes for a series of replicate trials several tests are possible:

(i) Test of agreement between the observed proportion of successes and the hypothetical p. This could take the form of a two-class goodness-of-fit test with one degree of freedom.

(ii) Goodness-of-fit test between the observed frequencies and the frequencies computed as $N(p + q)^n$ where p is the *observed* value. There would be $(n + 1)$ classes for comparison and in the absence of grouping there would be $(n + 1) - 2 = (n - 1)$ degrees of freedom for the test.

(iii) Goodness-of-fit test between the observed frequencies and the expected frequencies computed using the *hypothetical* p value. This would be testing *both* of the hypotheses tested seperately in (i) and (ii) above, and would have n degrees of freedom, i.e. the sum of the numbers of the other two tests.

Problems

6–1   A genetics class examined the *Drosophila* population resulting from the crossing of heterozygous females, w/ + with w/y males, the recessive mutant gene w (white-eyed) being sex-linked. The ratio of red-eyed (wild type) to white-eyed (mutants) was expected to be $1:1$. The numbers actually counted were: red-eyed 768 and white-eyed 818. Examine the goodness-of-fit of the observed to the expected frequencies.

6-2 In another class, the population of *Drosophila* resulting from crosses of the form ♀(vg/+)×(vg/+) ♂ (in a heterozygous F_1 population) was examined. The mutant gene vg (vestigial-winged) is recessive so the ratio of wild type (fully-winged) to vestigial-winged was expected to be $3:1$. The numbers actually counted were: fully-winged 2492 and vestigial-winged 664. Examine the goodness-of-fit between the observed and expected frequencies.

6-3 Complete the analysis of the data of Problem 4-7 by testing the goodness-of-fit of the observed to expected frequencies. Does the test lead to the same conclusion as the tests completed earlier?

6-4 Complete the analysis of the data of Problem 4-8 by testing the goodness-of-fit of the observed to expected frequencies. Does the test lead to the same conclusion as the tests completed earlier?

6-5 Complete the analysis of the data of Problem 5-4 by testing the goodness-of-fit of the observed to expected frequencies. Does the test lead to the same conclusion as the tests completed earlier?

7 Analysis of Frequencies: Double Classification

7.1 Association of attributes: 2×2 tables

In our analysis of frequencies so far (Chapter 6) we have considered cases in which observations have been classified according to one set of criteria only. It frequently happens however that we apply two or more classifications to the same population. In such cases it is possible not only to test agreement with hypotheses related to each classification but also to test for the independence between simultaneous classifications, i.e. to test for association. We will consider first the simplest case in which there are two classifications each into two mutually exclusive categories, and there are no hypotheses relating to the classifications individually.

As part of a study of laterality in man, the association between handedness and eye dominance was investigated. 400 school children were classified into left-handed or right-handed, and left-eye-dominant or right-eye-dominant. The results were as follows:

		Left-handed	Right-handed	(Total)
Left-eyed	Observed	27	110	(137)
	Expected	18.5 $(+8.5)$	118.5 (-8.5)	
Right-eyed	Observed	27	236	(263)
	Expected	35.5 (-8.5)	227.5 $(+8.5)$	
	(Total)	(54)	(346)	(400)

Although there are no hypotheses leading to particular expected frequencies from the individual classifications, on the null hypothesis of independence between the classifications there are expected values for each of the four resulting categories. For example, as 54 children were left-handed and 137 left-eyed, the number of children expected to be *both* left-handed and left-eyed is $(54 \times 137)/400 = 18.495$, rounded to 18.5. Corresponding expected values can be calculated similarly for all four categories. A goodness-of-fit test is now possible, with four comparisons, thus:

$$\chi^2 = \frac{8.5^2}{18.5} + \frac{(-8.5)^2}{118.5} + \frac{(-8.5)^2}{35.5} + \frac{8.5^2}{227.5} = \underline{6.868}$$

It might appear that the value of χ^2 would have three degrees of freedom (one less than the number of comparisons) but the expected values were computed from the observed frequencies (the marginal totals) and two degrees of freedom were thereby lost, leaving only *one degree of freedom*. Note that once the marginal totals have been fixed a single observed frequency inserted in one cell of the table will determine all the others. With only one degree of freedom the correction for continuity (see § 6.2) should be applied. This takes the form of reducing the magnitude of all four deviations by 0.5 before squaring. In practice we do not normally compute the four contributions in this way but employ the derived formula, below. For a 2 × 2 table:

	A_1	A_2	*(Total)*
B_1	a	b	$(a+b)$
B_2	c	d	$(c+d)$
(Total)	$(a+c)$	$(b+d)$	$(a+b+c+d) = n$

:it may be shown that:

$$\sum \frac{(O - E)^2}{E} = \frac{n(ad - bc)^2}{(a+c)(b+d)(a+b)(c+d)}$$

and with the correction for continuity:

$$\chi^2_{corr} = \frac{n(|ad - bc|^* - \frac{1}{2}n)^2}{(a+c)(b+d)(a+b)(c+d)}, \text{ with one degree of freedom}$$

For the above example we have:

$$\chi^2_{corr} = \frac{400(27 \times 236 - 27 \times 110 - 200)^2}{137 \times 263 \times 54 \times 346} = \underline{6.09} \text{ , with one degree of freedom, giving } P < 0.05$$

The test shows significant association between the two classifications and as the observed number of left-handed and left-eyed children exceeded that expected we conclude that, in the population represented by our sample of 400, left-handed children tend to be left-eye-dominant.

7.2   Differences between proportions and percentages

The 2 × 2 table can be applied to what may at first seem a very different

* $|ad - bc|$ denotes the positive difference between the two products.

kind of problem, the test of significance between two samples assessed in terms of the number of observations falling into one or other of two mutually exclusive classes, the problem of section 4.5.

The lawn of Problem 4–2 had been treated with selective herbicide several weeks previously. Another similar area of lawn had been left untreated as a control. This area was sampled with 300 random point-quadrats and 105 hits were recorded, indicating 35% cover of daisies. In order to compare the two percentages, i.e. 25% and 35%, we need to use the raw data in terms of hits and misses, thus:

	Lawn 1 (treated)	Lawn 2 (control)	(Total)
Hits	50	105	(155)
Misses	150	195	(345)
(Total)	(200)	(300)	(500)

$$\chi^2_{corr} = \frac{500(150 \times 105 - 50 \times 195 - 250)^2}{155 \times 345 \times 200 \times 300} = \underline{5.15} \text{, with one degree of}$$

freedom, giving
$P < 0.05$

We conclude that the cover percentage of daisies in the treated lawn is significantly different from that in the control. It might be argued that as the herbicide is not likely to *increase* daisy cover a 'one-tailed' test is appropriate and $P < 0.025$. Note that as frequencies are used in the test comparisons between treatments should be made before reduction of the results to percentages.

7.3   Association of attributes: $c \times r$ tables

Tests of association (see § 7.1) and comparisons of proportions and percentages (see §7.2) can be extended to the more general c (columns) $\times r$ (rows) table. The derived formula for the 2×2 table is not applicable so we normally use the general formula for χ^2 and compute $\Sigma[(O - E)^2/E]$. The number of degrees of freedom available for testing association is $(c - 1)(r - 1)$, and since this exceeds unity for all tables larger than 2×2 the correction for continuity is not applied. Interpretation of association demonstrated by means of a 2×2 table is often quite straight forward as it is either simply positive or negative. Significant association in the larger ($c \times r$) tables however, is frequently more complex and difficult to interpret (see § 8.2) and it is an advantage to have available for inspection the $(O - E)$ term for each cell of the table as a guide to the sign and magnitude of the deviation. Where the test is being used to check the absence of association and the $(O - E)$ terms are unlikely to be needed another form of computation of χ^2 may be used, i.e. $\chi^2 = \Sigma(O^2/E) - n$. For the larger tables objection to low expected frequencies (< 5) decreases as the likelihood of an inflated contribution from an individual cell influencing the final total χ^2 is reduced. Provided that expected frequencies do not fall below unity and only a small proportion are less than five, the conclusions drawn from the analysis are likely to be reliable.

In a project to examine the relationship between eye colour and defects in vision 878 children were classified into five categories on eye colour and independently into three categories according to whether they had normal, short, or long sight. The results can be analysed by means of a 3×5 table, thus:

Eye colour		Normal	Short	Long	(Total)
Blue	O E	268 255.44 $+12.56$	75 84.74 -9.74	13 15.81 -2.81	(356)
Green	O E	75 80.36 -5.36	32 26.66 $+5.34$	5 4.97 $+0.03$	(112)
Grey	O E	92 93.28 -1.28	30 30.95 -0.95	8 5.77 $+2.23$	(130)
Hazel	O E	75 81.80 -6.80	33 27.14 $+5.86$	6 5.06 $+0.94$	(114)
Brown	O E	120 119.11 $+0.89$	39 39.51 -1.51	7 7.37 -0.37	(166)
(Total)		(630) (0.01)	(209) (0.00)	(39) (0.02)	(878)

$$\chi^2 = \frac{12.56^2}{255.44} + \frac{9.74^2}{84.74} + \frac{2.81^2}{15.81} + \frac{5.36^2}{80.36} + \frac{5.34^2}{26.66} + \frac{0.03^2}{4.97} + \text{etc.}$$

$\underline{= 6.61}$, with $(3-1)(5-1) =$ eight degrees of freedom, giving $P > 0.5$

The conclusion then is that no significant association has been demonstrated. (For a $c \times r$ table with significant association see § 8.2.)

7.4   Test of homogeneity

The size or an individual experiment is often severely limited by availability of living material, extent of culture facilities, or the time needed to carry out the operations involved. Investigators frequently wish to amalgamate data from several similar experiments and draw conclusions from all available evidence. Before this is done it is desirable to check the consistency of results between experiments, i.e. to check that the data are homogeneous. Even when it is possible to carry out a large experiment or survey it is often wise to plan it in replicate sections so as to provide a check on technique. We will be concerned here only with data in the form of frequencies: the parallel situation with measurement data can be dealt with using the methods of Chapter 10.

If we are not concerned to test agreement with hypothetical frequencies we have only to test the hypothesis of no-association between the classification into categories *within* experiments and classification *between* experiments. For this we need only the methods of sections 7.1 and 7.3. In the course of some work on the autotropism of fungal spores, the germination patterns of touching spore pairs were classified into three categories, thus:

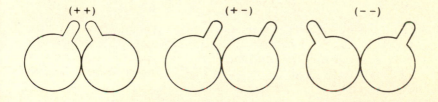

Because all observations on a particular batch of material had to be completed within about ten minutes the maximum number of spore pairs that could be found, classified and recorded proved to be about 200. It was desired to total the results for three such experiments. The results were as follows:

| Experiment | Germination pattern | | | |
	(+ +)	(+ −)	(− −)	(Total)
1	36	88	76	(200)
2	32	82	86	(200)
3	40	94	66	(200)
(Total)	(108)	(264)	(228)	(600)

The expected values are first calculated from the marginal totals, and as the row totals are all equal the expected frequencies for the three germination patterns are the same for each experiment: $200 \times 108/600 = 36$ for $(+ +)$, 88 for $(+ -)$ and 76 for $(- -)$. Giving,

$$\chi^2 = \frac{0^2 + 4^2 + 4^2}{36} + \frac{0^2 + 6^2 + 6^2}{88} + \frac{0^2 + 10^2 + 10^2}{76} = \frac{32}{36} + \frac{72}{88} + \frac{200}{76}$$

$$= \quad \underline{4.34}, \text{ with } (3-1)(3-1) = \text{four degrees of freedom, giving } P > 0.1$$

Deviations from expectation are therefore not significant and the data for the three experiments may be totalled for interpretation.

7.5   Combined test of homogeneity and goodness-of-fit

Although the observed frequencies in the above example were used to generate a causal hypothesis no existing hypothesis was under test when the experiments were carried out. When we have a hypothesis linking the observed frequencies within a single experiment, and for the data as a whole, we need to test both for homogeneity and agreement with hypothesis. Homogeneity could be tested as before but it is usually more efficient to obtain an estimate of the corresponding χ^2 (often called the 'heterogeneity χ^2' because it results from lack of homogeneity) by difference.

A genetics class examined the *Drosophila* population resulting from crosses between flies heterozygous for a recessive colour mutant. A ratio of 3:1 between wild-type and mutant phenotypes was expected. The population was scored in five batches by individual students and the results assembled for analysis, thus:

Batch	Wild-type			Mutant			(Total)
	O	E	Diff	O	E	Diff	
1	60	64.5	− 4.5	26	21.5	+ 4.5	(86)
2	75	81.0	− 6.0	33	27.0	+ 6.0	(108)
3	81	74.25	+ 6.75	18	24.75	− 6.75	(99)
4	70	84.0	−14.0	42	28.0	+14.0	(112)
5	54	56.25	− 2.25	21	18.75	+ 2.25	(75)
(Total)	(340)	(360)	(−20.00)	(140)	(120)	(+20.00)	(480)

First test the goodness-of-fit of the population totals to those expected on the hypothesis of a 3:1 ratio, thus:

$$\chi^2, \text{ for overall segregation} = \frac{(340 - 360)^2}{360} + \frac{(140 - 120)^2}{120}$$

$$= 4.444, \text{ with one degree of freedom,}$$
$$\text{giving } P < 0.05$$

So a significant overall departure from expectation is indicated. Now compute the χ^2 value for the goodness-of-fit of the observed frequencies in each batch to the 3:1 ratio, and then total these to give a total χ^2 value, thus:

Batch 1 $\chi^2 = (-4.5)^2/64.5$ $+$ $4.5^2/21.5$ $= 1.256$
Batch 2 $\chi^2 = (-6.0)^2/81.0$ $+$ $6.0^2/27.0$ $= 1.778$ all with
Batch 3 $\chi^2 = 6.75^2/74.25$ $+ (-6.75)^2/24.75 = 2.455$ one degree
Batch 4 $\chi^2 = (-14.0)^2/84.0$ $+$ $14.0^2/28.0$ $= 9.333$ of freedom
Batch 5 $\chi^2 = (-2.25)^2/56.25 +$ $2.25^2/18.75$ $= 0.360$

Total χ^2 $= 15.182$, with five degrees of freedom.

Obtain the heterogeneity χ^2 by subtraction and display the results in tabular form, thus:

Sources of variation	Degrees of freedom	χ^2	Probability
Deviation from 3:1 ratio	1	4.444	< 0.05
Heterogeneity	4	10.738	< 0.05
(Total)	(5)	(15.182)	

In the presence of significant heterogeneity we must question the meaning of the overall deviation from the 3:1 ratio. We re-examine the results for the individual batches and note:

(i) The deviation for batch 4 is outstandingly large, with an individual χ^2 value of 9.333, with one degree of freedom, which corresponds to $P < 0.01$.

(ii) No other batch shows significant deviation, all other χ^2 values being < 3.84, which corresponds to $P = 0.05$.

Investigation reveals that student No. 4 has defective colour vision and that the sorting of batch 4 is unreliable. As the material of batch 4 has been disposed of it cannot be re-sorted, so the data for this batch are deleted and the remainder re-analysed. (Problem 7–3.) (NB The discarding of aberrant data in this way is only justified if evidence other than that provided by the analysis shows it to be erroneous.)

7.6   Test of linkage

We have now met two kinds of situation which may be represented by a 2×2 or, more generally, by a $c \times r$ table. In one we were concerned only to examine association or lack of independence (see § 7.1 to 7.4) and in the other we were concerned also to test agreement between one set of marginal totals with a hypothesis (see § 7.5). In a $c \times r$ table we have a total of $(cr - 1)$ degrees of freedom, $(c - 1)(r - 1)$ of these are available for testing association, $(c - 1)$ for testing the agreement of column totals and $(r - 1)$ for testing the agreement of row totals to expected hypothetical values. There is a third kind of situation in which we use all these degrees of freedom. It arises when we are examining the pattern of segregation of two gene pairs.

Doubly heterozygous maize (*Zea mays*) plants were backcrossed with the double recessive. Four kinds of offspring resulted, with the following frequencies:

Red pericarp/not dwarf	PD	204
Red pericarp/dwarf	Pd	153
Colourless pericarp/not dwarf	pD	154
Colourless pericarp/dwarf	pd	165
		(676)

On the hypothesis of independent segregation the expected frequencies would be equal and 169. We first test the goodness-of-fit to this expectation. We could use the general formula, $\chi^2 = \Sigma[(O - E)^2/E]$, but as the expected value is the same throughout we use the simple form:

$$\chi^2 = \Sigma(O^2/E) - n, \text{ thus:}$$

$$\chi^2 = \frac{204^2 + 153^2 + 154^2 + 165^2}{169} - 676 = \underline{10.189} \text{ , with three degrees of freedom}$$

This corresponds to $P < 0.05$, indicating a significant departure from expectation. We do not know, however, whether this is due to departure from the $1:1$ ratio in the segregation P–p, or segregation D–d, or because the segregations are not independent, i.e. because of linkage. In order to resolve this we partition the χ^2 and make *three* comparisons each with one degree of freedom. Display the data in the form a 2×2 table.

	P	p	(*Total*)
D	204 (*a*)	154 (*b*)	(*a + b*)
d	153 (*c*)	165 (*d*)	(*c + d*)
(Total)	(*a + c*)	(*b + d*)	(*a + b + c + d*) = *n*

For the segregation $P - p$, we test the goodness-of-fit of $(a + c)$ and $(b + d)$ to the ratio $1:1$ by calculating:

$$\chi^2 = \frac{[(a + c) - (b + d)]^2}{n} = 2.136$$

For the segregation $D - d$

$$\chi^2 = \frac{[(a + b) - (c + d)]^2}{n} = 2.366$$

For the linkage:

$$\chi^2 = \frac{[(a + d) - (b + c)]^2}{n} = 5.686$$

Expressed in tabular form:

Sources of variation	Degrees of freedom	χ^2	P
Segregation $P - p$	1	2.136	> 0.1
Segregation $D - d$	1	2.366	> 0.1
Linkage	1	5.686	< 0.05
(Total)	(3)	(10.188)	

This leads us to the conclusion that deviation from $1:1$ expectation is not significant but that there is significant linkage between P and D, and p and d.

When $F_1 \times F_1$ crosses are made, the Mendelian expectation is $9:3:3:1$. The same kind of analysis is possible but the expressions used for calculating the individual χ^2 are as follows (using the same nomenclature as in the last example).

For the segregation P–p:

$$\chi^2 = \frac{1}{3n}[(a + c) - 3(b + d)]^2$$

For the segregation D–d:

$$\chi^2 = \frac{1}{3n}[(a + b) - 3(c + d)]^2$$

For the linkage:

$$\chi^2 = \frac{1}{9n}[(a + 9d) - 3(b + c)]^2$$

In our use of χ^2 in the examination of frequency data subject to double classification we have met an important new idea. We have seen how total variation corresponding to several degrees of freedom can be analysed to permit us to make selected comparisons corresponding to individual degrees of freedom. We do this by partitioning χ^2. In the final chapters of this book we shall see how to analyse variation in measurement data according to its several causes by partitioning sums-of-squares in the *analysis of variance*.

7.7 Alternative methods

In Chapters 6 and 7 so far we have used several different mathematical expressions to compute quantities which have then been compared with tabulated critical values of χ^2. These methods involve only simple arithmetic and have been employed successfully for many years but they do have several disadvantages. The computation of $\Sigma\chi^2$ for a $c \times r$ table, although simple, is tedious in that all the expected frequencies must first be calculated from the marginal totals. Although we have seen how, as in section 7.5, the heterogeneity χ^2 can be estimated by difference the value obtained is not identical to that computed directly, i.e. the values as computed are not strictly additive. The heterogeneity χ^2 computed for the example of section 7.5 by the method of sections 7.1 to 7.4 is 9.744 and not 10.738 as found by difference.

In recent years a different kind of solution has been developed and is well described in SOKAL and ROHLF (1969 and 1973). Although logarithmic functions are employed the increase in availability of electronic calculators may place the corresponding methods in a competitive position. They have several advantages: the computed quantities are strictly additive and in general fit more closely the theoretical χ^2 distribution: expected frequencies for $c \times r$ tables are not required. There are several methods of computation and the relevant tables of $f \log_e f$ and $(f + \frac{1}{2}) \log_e (f + \frac{1}{2})$ are included in both SOKAL and ROHLF (1973) and ROHLF and SOKAL (1969), but for the most efficient solutions a calculator with a $\log_e$ facility (and an accumulating memory) is required. The simple rules are, briefly:

Goodness-of-fit: Evaluate $2\,\Sigma O \ln \left(\dfrac{O}{E} \right)$ for all classes, where ln denotes '$\log_e$'. Apply the correction for continuity (by *reducing* deviations by 0.5) when there is one degree of freedom. The rules for lower limits of expected frequencies and for numbers of degrees of freedom as in Chapter 6.

Example: data of section 6.3.

$$\chi^2 = 2\left[315\ln\frac{315}{312.75} + 108\ln\frac{108}{104.25} + 101\ln\frac{101}{104.25} + 32\ln\frac{32}{34.75} \right]$$

$$= 2(2.2581 + 3.8167 - 3.1988 - 2.6382)$$
$$= \underline{0.4754} \ \ (\text{cf. } 0.470 \text{ of section } 6.3)$$

$c \times r$ *tables*:

(i) Compute and sum terms of the form $f \ln f$ for all the $c \times r$ observed frequencies, and for the grand total.

(ii) Compute and sum terms of the form $f \ln f$ for all $c + r$ marginal totals.

(iii) Compute 2 (i − ii).

Rules for lower limits of expected frequencies and for numbers of degrees of freedom as in section 7.3.

Example: data of section 7.4.

(i) $36\ln 36 + 88\ln 88 + 76\ln 76 + 32\ln 32 + \ldots \ldots \ldots \text{etc} \ldots \ldots$
$$\ldots 66\ln 66 + 600\ln 600 = 6396.7763$$

(ii) $108\ln 108 + 264\ln 264 + 228\ln 228 + 200\ln 200 + 200\ln 200 +$
$$200\ln 200 = 6394.6020$$

(iii) $2 \,(\text{i} - \text{ii}) = \underline{4.3486} \ \ (\text{cf. } 4.34 \text{ of § } 7.4)$

Problems

7–1 During a study of small-scale heterogeneity of agricultural grassland casual observation suggested that the presence of white clover (*Trifolium repens*) was associated with the casting activity of earthworms. To test this hypothesis a grid of 10×40 contiguous area samples, each 25 cm square, was marked out. The presence or absence of clover and of fresh worm casts was recorded for each sample. Of the 400 samples clover was present in a total of 260, casts in a total of 115, and *both* clover and casts were present in 90. Test the hypothesis of association.

7–2 A biology class had to be divided for practical work into two parts and taught by different members of staff in two different laboratories. At the time of the examination doubts were raised on the equality of opportunity which had been offered to the two groups of students. Their examination results are summarized below: examine them for heterogeneity.

	< 30	30–39	40–49	50–59	60–69	⩾ 70
Group A	3	8	32	18	12	5
Group B	6	12	22	12	8	3

7–3 Complete the analysis for the data of section 7.5 after deleting the data for batch 4.

7–4 A student investigated the effect of modifying experimentally the vaginal pH of mouse (*Mus musculus*) on the sex ratio of offspring and obtained the following results:

Treatment	Male	Female
Control (untreated)	34	31
pH 7.0	22	16
pH 4.0	9	21
pH 9.2	21	7

Analyse these data by the method of section 7.5.

7-5 An F_2 population of morning glory (*Pharbitis*) segregating for two genes Gg and Hh was found to consist of the following: GH 123, Gh 30, gH 27, and gh 21, giving a total of 201. Examine the segregation of each gene pair and test for linkage using the method of section 7.6.

7-6 Re-analyse the data of section 7.5 using the methods in section 7.7.

8 Interrelationships of Quantitative Variables

8.1 Kinds of information and relationships

There are two main kinds of information that we may have about a series of individuals or samples. One kind consists of measurements, counts, scores, etc., which take the form of a numerical assessment. We call this *quantitative* information. The other kind consists of a classification of the individuals or samples into a series of qualitatively different categories. We call this *qualitative* information. We can examine interrelationships for any of the three possible combinations thus, qualitative/qualitative, qualitative/quantitative, and quantitative/quantitative. As we shall see, in practice, the situation is more complex because the categories used in the qualitative classification may form a semi-quantitative series. Again, even when a numerical assessment is not made, it may still be possible to arrange the individuals or samples in order on the basis of a particular criterion, i.e. to rank them.

8.2 Qualitative/qualitative data

Interrelationship based on qualitative information is usually called *association* and examined by means of a $c \times r$ table as described in Chapter 7. We calculate χ^2 with $(c-1)(r-1)$ degrees of freedom and this permits us to test the association for significance. The χ^2 value itself is not a good measure of the closeness of association as its magnitude depends on the total number of observations. To compare the levels of association for two tables with the same number of degrees of freedom we use χ^2/n, the 'mean-square contingency'. The value of χ^2 does not indicate the nature of the association, e.g. for a 2×2 table whether the association is positive or negative. This must be discovered by examination of the table, from the sign and magnitude of one or more $(O-E)$ terms. It is possible, and sometimes necessary, to extend this type of treatment to situations in which the information is semi-quantitative in that the individuals or samples are classified into a number of classes which cover in a stepwise manner the range of some particular kind of variation, e.g. 'no symptom', 'slight symptoms', 'severe symptoms', 'dead', but the method is often unsatisfactory. Large numbers of observations are required and the interpretation of significant association (when demonstrated) is frequently difficult. An example of the successful application of the method follows.

During an autecological study of a particular woodland moss the relationship between the occurrence of the moss and the depth of raw-humus layer on the soil surface was examined. The moss, where present, was seen to grow either vigorously excluding other species and forming a pure weft, or less vigorously and to contribute along with several other species to a loose mixed weft. It was decided to utilize this natural discontinuity in the behaviour of the moss and thus avoid the practical problems of full quantification. Three classes were recognized: 0 = moss absent; 1 = moss present in mixed weft; 2 = moss present in pure weft. The depth of raw-humus was then arbitrarily scored: $0 < 1$ cm; $1 = 1-2$ cm; and $2 > 2$ cm. Three hundred random samples, each 25 cm × 25 cm, were examined and records made of moss occurrence and raw-humus depth, using the classes defined above. The results were entered into a 3 × 3 table, thus:

Humus			Moss					(Total)
			0		1		2	
0	O	36	+8.2	15	−2.8	7	−5.4	(58)
	E	27.8		17.8		12.4		
1	O	65	−5.1	37	−7.8	44	+12.9	(146)
	E	70.1		44.8		31.1		
2	O	43	−3.1	40	+10.6	13	−7.5	(96)
	E	46.1		29.4		20.5		
(Total)		(144)		(92)		(64)		(300)

$$\chi^2 = \frac{8.2^2}{27.8} + \frac{2.8^2}{17.8} + \frac{5.4^2}{12.4} + \frac{5.1^2}{70.1} + \frac{7.8^2}{44.8} + \frac{12.9^2}{31.1} + \frac{3.1^2}{46.1} + \frac{10.6^2}{29.4} + \frac{7.5^2}{20.5}$$
$$= 2.419 + 0.440 + 2.352 + 0.371 + 1.358 + 5.351 + 0.208 + 3.822 + 2.744$$
$$= \underline{19.065}, \text{ with four degrees of freedom, giving } P < 0.001$$

Highly significant departure from random expectation having been established, examination of the sign and magnitude of differences for individual cells of the table revealed that:

(i) Pure wefts tend to occur on the intermediate depth of raw-humus (+12.9).

(ii) Mixed wefts tend to occur on deep raw-humus (+10.6).

(iii) The moss tends to be absent from shallow raw-humus (+8.2).

These results suggested the hypothesis that the moss tends to colonize the soil surface when the remains of other species have accumulated to form a little raw humus, that it then grows vigorously, forming a dense pure weft but by its own growth brings about a further increase in depth of the raw-humus and renders its habitat less suitable for itself. Its vigour then appears to fall and other species invade to produce a mixed weft. Microscopic examination of raw-humus profiles showed stratification of plant remains which supported this hypothesis.

8.3   Qualitative/quantitative data

We are frequently called upon to examine the relationship between a qualitative classification on the one hand and the level of some quantitative variable on the other. In fact, this is the normal situation arising from an experiment with two or more qualitatively different treatments and the response quantitatively assessed. In ecological work the qualitative classification may rest simply on the presence or absence of a particular species in a sample and the quantitative variable may be the level of an environmental factor. The method is to sort the individuals or samples into their qualitatively different classes, calculate the mean value of the quantitative variable for each class, and examine the difference or differences between the means for significance using an appropriate test. When there are only two classes we can use the t-tests of sections 3.2 and 3.3. When there are more than two classes the t-test is inappropriate and the methods of Chapters 9 and 10 are called for.

8.4   Quantitative/quantitative data

Two sets of quantitative data relating to a single series of individuals or samples are met with in a number of different biological situations resulting from both surveys and experiments. The method of analysis to be used may depend on the origin and form of the data, the objective of the investigator, or both. When we have quantitative data on two attributes, X and Y say, for a series of individuals (i.e. a sample) from a population we may need to address ourselves to several questions concerning the *parent population*.

(i) Do X and Y vary independently or are they related?
If they appear to be related. . . .

(ii) What is the form of their relationship, e.g. does it tend to be rectilinear or curvilinear?
If substantially rectilinear. . . .

(iii) Is the relationship positive or negative, and how close to an exact rectilinear relationship is it ?

(iv) What is the equation of the line to which the relationship tends?

(v) To what extent can we account for the variation in Y (say) in terms of the observed variation in X, and how reliably can we predict values of Y from observed values of X?
In practice it is wise to begin the examination of such data by plotting a

point or *scatter* diagram, using two axes at right-angles to represent the two variables. Such a diagram will often reveal whether:

(a) X and Y are related or independent,

(b) any relationship is recti- or curvi-linear, and

(c) if it is positive or negative.

When we take a random sample from a population and measure some quantitative attribute of each individual we usually find that the measurements tend to be normally distributed (see § 2.2). When we measure two such attributes both sets of measurements tend to be normally distributed and the data may be described as bivariate-normal. In the same way that a normal distribution may be represented by a bell-shaped curve so a bivariate-normal distribution may be represented by a domed surface.

8.5   Correlation

When we have a set of bivariate-normal data in which X and Y appear, from a scatter diagram, to be related and the relationship appears to be rectilinear we may wish to assess the closeness of the apparent relationship and test its significance at population level. This may be done by using the method of correlation. We need a measure of the degree to which X and Y vary together. One such measure is the sum of the products of the joint deviations of X and Y from their respective means, divided by the number of degrees of freedom, i.e. the covariance (C) between X and Y, thus: $C_{XY} = \Sigma(X - \overline{X})(Y - \overline{Y})/(N - 1)$. The covariance is positive when X and Y tend to vary together and negative when one tends to increase as the other decreases, but it is not a suitable measure of the closeness of the relationship because (like a variance) its magnitude depends on the units in which X and Y are measured. This disadvantage is removed by expressing the deviation in standard deviation units. The resulting quantity is called the *product-moment correlation coefficient* and our estimate of it (from a sample) is designated r, thus:

$$r = \frac{1}{N-1} \sum \left(\frac{(X - \overline{X})}{s_X} \frac{(Y - \overline{Y})}{s_Y} \right) = \frac{\Sigma(X - \overline{X})(Y - \overline{Y})}{\sqrt{[\Sigma(X - \overline{X})^2 \Sigma(Y - \overline{Y})^2]}}$$

Or, in a form more suitable for computation from the raw data:

$$r = \frac{\Sigma XY - (\Sigma X \, \Sigma Y/N)}{\sqrt{[(\Sigma X^2 - (\Sigma X)^2/N)(\Sigma Y^2 - (\Sigma Y)^2/N)]}}$$

$\Sigma(X - \overline{X})(Y - \overline{Y})$ is known as the sum-of-products of X and Y and is denoted by Σxy, so

$$r = \frac{\Sigma xy}{\sqrt{(\Sigma x^2 \Sigma y^2)}}$$

The coefficient r can have values ranging from $+1$ to -1. $r = +1$ corresponds to a rectilinear relationship (of the form $Y = a + bX$) in which the two variables are positively related. $r = -1$ corresponds to a rectilinear relationship in which the two variables are negatively related. Values of r near $+1$ and -1 indicate an approach to a rectilinear relationship, for which the bivariate-normal surface would take the form of a narrow ridge rather than a dome. Intermediate values of r may be due to absence of a relationship or to the existence of a relationship which is not essentially rectilinear. Such values should only be interpreted with the aid of a scatter diagram. (See Fig. 8–1.)

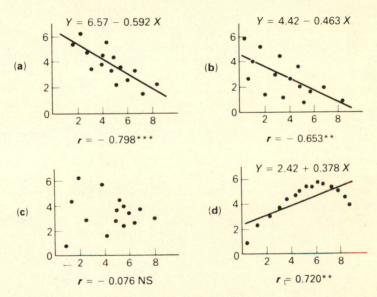

Fig. 8–1 Samples from four bivariate distributions plotted as scatter diagrams with computed r values, and results of regression analyses were linear component significant.

Although the sample correlation coefficient provides a measure of correlation it does not directly indicate the level of significance of the relationship at population level. When N is small there is a real possibility of obtaining a value of r deviating markedly from zero because of accidental 'covariation' in the few pairs of values involved. We can test the significance of the deviation of r from zero by evaluating the ratio $r/(\text{S.E. of } r)$ and equating this to t with $(N-2)$ degrees of freedom. The number of degrees of freedom is $(N-2)$ because both r and t have been estimated from the data. The S.E. of the estimate of r depends only on r and N and is $\sqrt{[(1-r^2)/(N-2)]}$. In practice we rarely need this test as tables have been prepared of the critical values of r. (See Table 3.)

During a search for suitable parameters for use in an investigation of the environmental factors controlling the 'performance' of Timothy grass (*Phleum pratense*) a number of vegetative and reproductive attributes were measured for a random sample of 30 flowering shoots from a population. Among these attributes were length of the uppermost leaf (including sheath) and length of the inflorescence spike. The results were as follows:

Shoot No.	1	2	3	4	5	6	7	8	9	10
Leaf (cm)	23.4	22.0	25.0	18.1	18.9	20.5	19.1	27.5	21.6	14.3
Spike (cm)	9.8	9.5	12.2	8.3	9.5	9.2	8.5	12.1	10.4	5.5
Shoot No.	11	12	13	14	15	16	17	18	19	20
Leaf	20.8	16.3	23.1	17.4	17.0	26.8	12.5	18.4	16.7	24.0
Spike	10.6	5.5	10.5	7.4	6.8	11.7	4.1	9.3	6.2	11.0
Shoot No.	21	22	23	24	25	26	27	28	29	30
Leaf	24.2	21.2	15.0	20.0	20.1	19.2	21.0	13.0	19.7	26.0
Spike	10.2	9.6	5.0	8.5	9.7	7.0	7.9	4.7	8.3	12.6

A scatter diagram, Fig. 8–2, indicated that these two attributes are positively related and that the relationship is substantially rectilinear. To permit comparison with relationships between other pairs of attributes an assessment of the closeness of this relationship was needed. As it is reasonable to assume a bivariate-normal distribution the method of correlation may be used and r calculated.

$$\Sigma X = 602.8 \qquad \Sigma Y = 261.6 \qquad N = 30$$
$$\Sigma X^2 = 12\,552.20 \qquad \Sigma Y^2 = 2438.16 \qquad \Sigma XY = 5503.44$$
$$\Sigma x^2 = 439.94 \qquad \Sigma y^2 = 157.01 \qquad \Sigma xy = 247.02$$

$$r = \frac{247.02}{\sqrt{(439.94 \times 157.01)}} = +0.940 \text{ with 28 degrees of freedom}$$

We can compute $t = \dfrac{0.940}{\sqrt{[(1-0.8836)/28]}} = 14.58$, with 28 degrees of freedom, giving $P < 0.001$

Referring the computed value of r to Table 3 leads to the same conclusion.

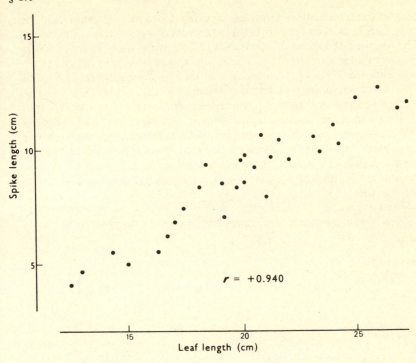

Fig. 8–2 Correlation between leaf length and spike length in Timothy grass (*Phleum pratense*).

8.6 Regression

The examination of a relationship by the method of correlation presupposes the data to be bivariate-normal. There are many situations in which this assumption is not justified, e.g. when the levels of one variable are controlled by the investigator as a series of treatments in an experiment. It is under just such circumstances that regression analysis, which answers a rather different set of questions, is particularly appropriate. In regression analysis we recognize the asymmetry of the relationship by distinguishing between the independent variable (e.g. causal factor) and the dependent variable (e.g. the possible response). The assumptions which we make in the analysis (which define the mathematical model) and therefore which should be fulfilled before it is applied are as follows:

(i) that the independent variable, X, is measured without error,

(ii) that for each value of X there is a corresponding 'true' value of Y such as to fit a rectilinear relationship between X and Y,

(iii) that the measurements of Y show random variation and are normally distributed about their 'true' mean, and

(iv) that the variance of the values of Y about their 'true' mean is the same for all values of X.

Unfortunately there is no simple way in which one can satisfy oneself that all of these assumptions are justified!

The equation of the straight line is of the form $Y = a + bX$, where b defines the gradient and a the point at which the line crosses the Y axis. The values of a and b must be estimated from the sample data so that the maximum amount of variation in Y is accounted for in terms of variation in X; or in other words, so that the variation in Y not accounted for is at a minimum. In the same way that we assess variation about a mean in terms of the sum of the squares of the deviations from the mean, so we assess the deviations from linear relationship in terms of the sum of the squares of the deviations from values predicted by the regression equation, i.e. from the regression line (Fig. 8–3).

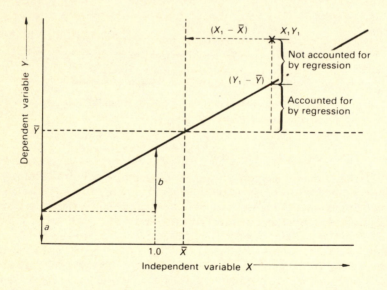

Fig. 8–3 Regression of Y upon X.

b is called the regression coefficient and is estimated by:

$$b = \frac{\Sigma(X - \overline{X})(Y - \overline{Y})}{\Sigma(X - \overline{X})^2} \equiv \frac{\Sigma XY - (\Sigma X)(\Sigma Y)/N}{\Sigma X^2 - (\Sigma X)^2/N} \equiv \frac{\Sigma xy}{\Sigma x^2}$$

a   which is called the 'intercept' is then estimated by substituting the computed value of *b* in the equation:

$$a = \bar{Y} - b\bar{X}$$

In order to plot the regression line two convenient values of X are selected (or three to provide a check) and the corresponding Y values computed from the regression equation. The regression line should not be drawn much beyond the range of the points for which it is computed as this would be unjustified extrapolation.

As with correlation it is usually best to begin an analysis by drawing a scatter diagram. The points cluster may be markedly linear or the points may be well spread. Where the tendency to linearity appears to be slight we need to test the significance of the regression, in other words to question whether the variation in Y accounted for by its regression on X in the sample is great enough for us to conclude that there is a linear relationship between X and Y in the parent population. In such cases it will be noted that the value of b is low and the regression line is far from being the line of optical-best-fit. In order to test the significance of the regression we analyse the variation of Y into two components, thus,:

$$\text{total variation in } Y \text{ (as sum-of-squares)} = \Sigma y^2$$

$$\text{variation accounted for by regression} = \frac{(\Sigma xy)^2}{\Sigma x^2}$$

$$\therefore \text{ variation } not \text{ accounted for} = \Sigma y^2 - \frac{(\Sigma xy)^2}{\Sigma x^2}$$

This may be converted to the variance not accounted for, the residual variance, by dividing by its number of degrees of freedom, $(N-2)$, thus:

$$\text{residual variance, } s_R{}^2 = \frac{1}{N-2}\left(\Sigma y^2 - \frac{(\Sigma xy)^2}{\Sigma x^2}\right)$$

One method of testing the significance of regression is to test whether the estimated value of b deviates significantly from zero (cf. significance test for r). We calculate $t = b/(\text{S.E. of } b)$, with $(N-2)$ degrees of freedom. The S.E. of b is $s_R/\sqrt{\Sigma x^2}$, so we compute $t = b\sqrt{(\Sigma x^2/s_R{}^2)}$. (An alternative method is described in section 9.6.)

Having established that regression on X accounts for a significant amount of the variation in Y, statements involving confidence limits may be called for. The 95% confidence limits of b are $b \pm t_{0.05} \times s_R/\sqrt{\Sigma x^2}$, where t has $(N-2)$ degrees of freedom. In the same way that we can attach confidence limits to a population mean (μ) estimated from a sample (as $\bar{X}$, see § 2.4 and 2.5) so we can attach confidence limits to the 'true' or population values of Y predicted for a particular value of X by means of the regression equation. Such limits, over the whole range of X, define the *confidence zone* of the regression line. There are two sources of error, one in the estimation of the Y population mean (at $\bar{X}$) and the other

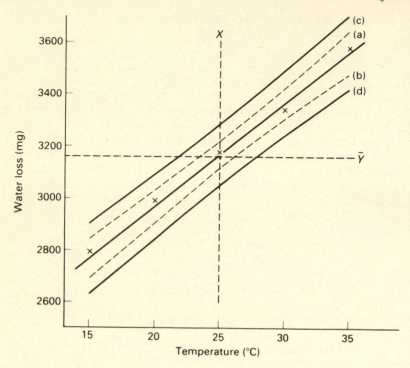

Fig. 8–4 Regression of water loss by mice on temperature, with 95% confidence zone of regression line (a) and (b), and 95% confidence limits of predictions of water loss from temperature for single groups of mice (c) and (d).

in the estimation of b. The effect of any error in the former is constant over the range of X but the effect of any error in b increases as values of X deviate from $\overline{X}$. We can allow for both these sources of error by computing the confidence limits: $\hat{Y} \pm t \times s_R \sqrt{[1/N + (X' - \overline{X})^2/\Sigma x^2]}$, where $\hat{Y}$ is the predicted Y value and X' the particular value of X for which the prediction is required. The confidence zone is narrowest at $X = \overline{X}$ and becomes wider for values both above and below this, Fig. 8–4a and b. Regression equations are frequently used to predict *individual* values of Y from values of X and the reliability of such predictions may be important. Predicted values for individuals are subject to an additional source of error – deviation from the regression line – and this is allowed for by computing the confidence limits for an *individual* predicted value of Y as $\hat{Y} \pm t \times s_R \sqrt{[1 + 1/N + (X' - \overline{X})^2/\Sigma x^2]}$, Fig. 8–4 c and d.

As part of an investigation on the effect of temperature variation on mice, the rate of water-loss by a group of mice was determined for a series of temperatures by absorbing the water evolved by the group in a particular time. The following results were obtained:

Temperature (°C)	15	20	25	30	35
Water evolved (mg)	2794	2924	3175	3340	3576

The temperature, which was controlled experimentally, becomes the independent variable X, and the amount of water evolved becomes the dependent variable Y. The scatter diagram, Fig. 8–4, shows that the sample values approach a rectilinear relationship so we compute the regression equation.

$$\Sigma X = 125 \qquad \Sigma Y = 15\,809 \qquad N = 5$$
$$\Sigma X^2 = 3375 \qquad \Sigma Y^2 = 50\,380\,213 \qquad \Sigma XY = 405\,125$$
$$\Sigma x^2 = 250 \qquad \Sigma y^2 = 395\,316.8 \qquad \Sigma xy = 9\,900$$
$$b = 9\,900/250 = 39.60$$
$$\overline{X} = 125/5, \overline{Y} = 15\,809/5 = 3161.8, \text{ so}$$
$$a = 3161.8 - (39.60 \times 25) = 2171.8$$

Equation becomes: $Y = 39.60\,X + 2172$

To plot the regression line let $X' = 15$, giving $\hat{Y} = 2766$, and let $X' = 35$, giving $\hat{Y} = 3558$. Plot points (15, 2766) and (35, 3558) and join them with a straight line.

To test the significance of regression compute the residual variance:

$$s_R^2 = \frac{1}{3}\left(395\,316.8 - \frac{9900^2}{250}\right) = 1092.3$$

then:

$$t = 39.6\sqrt{(250/1092.3)} = \underline{18.945}, \text{ with three degrees of freedom,}$$
$$\text{giving } P < 0.001$$

To obtain values for plotting 95% confidence zone:

$$t_{0.05} \text{ for three degrees of freedom} = 3.182$$
$$s_R = \sqrt{1092.3} = 33.05$$

Substituting for X', 15 or 35

$$95\% \text{ limits (at } \overline{X} \pm 10) \text{ are } \hat{Y} \pm 3.182 \times 33.051\sqrt{(1/5 + 100/250)}$$
$$\pm 81.5$$

and similarly for other values of X'.

The usefulness of linear regression is greatly increased by transformation. When bivariate data are plotted as a scatter diagram the relationship may appear clearly curvilinear. Consideration of the shape of the points cluster and/or the kind of relationship being studied will often suggest a simple form of transformation which when applied to one or both variables would convert their relationship to rectilinear form. Re-plotting the data after transformation will usually show whether transformation has been effective. Where log transformation of one or both variables is suggested computation may be avoided at this stage by using log or semi-log graph paper. When an apparently effective transformation has been found the analysis of the relationship can usually be completed as a straightforward linear regression. In linear regression we assume that the error variance of the dependent variable, Y, is the same for all values of the independent variable, X. If this is true for the original data it *cannot* be true for the transformed data, and vice versa. Fortunately, data transformation, when called for, usually has the effect of making the error variance homogeneous. (see SOKAL and ROHLF (1969) section 14.12. or (1973) section 11.7.)

In the form of regression analysis which we have been considering, which we might now refer to as 'Model 1', an important assumption has been that the independent variable, X, is measured without error. Not infrequently we need to investigate relationships in which this assumption is not justified. Suppose we wish to investigate the relationship between the heights of trees, Y, and the availability of phosphorus from the soil, X. We cannot measure X directly, but only estimate it by chemical analysis of extracts from soil samples collected within the trees' rooting zone. Although the chemical determinations may be made with precision as estimates of X they will be subject to substantial error. Such situations require a different form of analysis known as 'Model 2' regression. Details will be found in SOKAL and ROHLF (1969) section 14.13 and Box 14.12.

Further regression topics are dealt with in section 9.6.

Problems

8–1   In an investigation of the relationship between body weight and lung capacity, LC, (estimated by spirometer) a student obtained the following results with a randomly selected group of Caucasian females between 17 and 19 years old.

Subject	1	2	3	4	5	6	7	8	9	10
Wt(Kg)	54.4	56.2	49.0	63.5	60.8	59.9	62.6	62.1	52.2	50.8
LC(1)	3.87	3.26	2.14	4.13	3.44	2.78	2.91	3.33	3.20	2.17
	11	12	13	14	15	16	17	18	19	20
	57.2	48.1	54.0	50.8	49.9	46.3	59.0	56.2	61.2	53.1
	3.13	2.47	3.03	2.88	2.65	2.03	3.21	3.45	3.61	2.53

Plot these results as a scatter diagram, examine the nature of the relationship and test its significance by computing the product-moment correlation coefficient, r.

8-2 In an experiment to examine the effect of glucose concentration in the medium on linear growth of *Geotrichum candidum* (a mould) the following results were obtained for a medium countaining mineral nutrients plus glucose at 50 mg 1^{-1}.

Days from inoculation	3	5	7	9	11	13
Radius of colony (mm)	7.7	13.0	17.5	23.0	26.7	29.7

Plot these results as a scatter diagram, examine the regression of colony diameter on time and attach 95% confidence limits to *b*, the linear growth rate.

8-3 During an investigation of the cause(s) of irregular growth in a plantation of Sitka spruce (*Picea sitchensis*), 40 trees were selected to cover the full height range within a certain forest plot. Each of the 40 trees was felled, its total height measured and the nutrient content of the needles of the leading shoot determined by chemical analysis. Assuming that the nitrogen concentration in the needles of the leading shoot estimates without error the level of availability of nitrogen compounds to the tree examine the regression of tree height in metres (Y) on the nitrogen content in percentage dry weight (X). Test the significance of regression, predict the tree height for 1.0% nitrogen and attach 95% confidence limits to the predicted height of an individual tree with this percentage nitrogen.

Summary of results:

$$\Sigma X = 40.92 \qquad \Sigma Y = 249.36 \qquad N = 40$$
$$\Sigma X^2 = 46.885 \qquad \Sigma Y^2 = 2038.25 \qquad \Sigma XY = 297.93$$

9 Analysis of Variance: Single Classification

9.1 Why do we need analysis of variance?

We have considered already (Chapter 3) how the difference between two sample means may be tested for significance. In practice we are often faced with the need to examine the differences between the means of more than two samples. On meeting this problem for the first time many biologists react by testing the significance of each difference separately by means of the t test. This is neither efficient nor proper.

That it is not proper can be understood by recalling the nature of a test of significance. When we apply such a test at, for example, the 5% level of significance there is a probability of 1 : 20 of our concluding that the two population means are different when in fact they are equal (i.e. of making a Type 1 error). This is so for each comparison we make and it may be calculated (as $1 - 0.95^{21}$) that for an experiment with 7 treatments, and hence 21 comparisons, there is a probability of 0.66 of making at least one Type 1 error. This is clearly not good enough. It would be possible by using, for instance, the 1% level of significance to reduce the probability but this would greatly increase the risk of rejecting as non-significant differences which were real (i.e. of making a Type 2 error). What is needed is a technique which examines the variation within the whole group of sample means. This is the technique of analysis of variance. That the use of multiple t tests is not efficient will become clear when the economy and elegance of the analysis of variance has been appreciated. The analysis is carried out in two steps:

(i) Test of the null hypothesis that the samples could have been drawn from a single population, or from several populations with equal means.

(ii) Comparisons between sample means.

9.2 Preliminary analysis

Despite its name, analysis of variance does not involve the analysis of variance itself but the partitioning of the total sum-of-squares (Σx^2) to provide several variance estimates which are then compared. In its simplest form it consists of a comparison between two estimates of the overall variance (of the complete set of measurements included in the analysis), one estimate being based on the variance of the sample means about the grand mean and the other based on the variance of the individual measurements about the sample means. If the null hypothesis were true we would expect the ratio of these two estimates (between-sample variance/within-sample variance) to approximate to unity. If, on the other hand, the sample means estimate different population means then we would expect the ratio to exceed unity. In practice we equate the ratio to the statistic F which enables us to estimate the probability of obtaining such a ratio (or one larger) if the null hypothesis were true. It will be recalled that in calculating a simple variance the sum of the squares of the deviations from the mean (i.e. the sum-of-squares, $\Sigma(X-\overline{X})^2$, $\Sigma X^2 - (\Sigma X)^2/N$, or Σx^2) is divided by the appropriate number of degrees of freedom $(N-1)$. In the analysis of variance we partition the total sum-of-squares according to the cause of the variation (e.g. differences between sample means and differences between replicate measurements in the same sample) and divide the two components by their numbers of degrees of freedom to obtain the corresponding variances. Conventionally these are called *mean-squares*. We then calculate the variance ratio as the ratio of the two mean squares and equate to F.

We have met already, in our use of t, a ratio in the form (difference)/(S.E. of difference) in which we have to take account of the number of degrees of freedom of the denominator. F is a ratio of two variances so both numerator and denominator have their own numbers of degrees of freedom. We have to take account of these when entering a calculated value in the table of F.

Consider the results of an experiment with k treatments and n replicates for each treatment. The results would have the form:

Treatments

	1	2	3	....	k	
Replicates	X_{11}	X_{21}	X_{31}	....	X_{k1}	
	X_{12}	X_{22}	X_{32}	....	X_{k2}	
		& etc. to ...				
	X_{1n}	X_{2n}	X_{3n}	...	X_{kn}	
Treatment totals	T_1	T_2	T_3	....	T_n	GT Grand total
Treatment means	X_1	X_1	X_3	....	X_n	$\overline{X}$ Grand mean

(i) Compute the *correction term* C as $(\mathrm{GT})^2/kn$ (This is the square of the sum of all values of X divided by the total number of values. It is equivalent to $(\Sigma X)^2/N$ in a variance calculation.)

(ii) Compute the total sum-of-squares, SS as $\Sigma X^2 - \mathrm{C}$ (This is Σx^2, the sum-of-squares in a variance calculation.)

(iii) Compute the *sum-of squares for between treatments*, SST, as

$\Sigma T^2/n - C$. (What is needed here is a sum-of-squares, based on treatment means or treatment totals, which when divided by the appropriate number of degrees of freedom will yield an estimate of overall variance. The sum-of-squares of treatment means about the grand mean would be given by $\Sigma \bar{X}^2 - (\Sigma \bar{X})^2/k$. The sum-of-squares of the individual values would be n times this, i.e. $n(\Sigma \bar{X}^2 - (\Sigma \bar{X})^2/k)$. Replacing means by totals this becomes $\Sigma T^2/n - C$.)

(iv) Compute the *sum-of-squares for error*, SSE, as $SS - SST$. (This could be computed directly as:

$$\Sigma X_1^2 - (\Sigma X_1)^2/n + \Sigma X_2^2 - (\Sigma X_2)^2/n + \ldots\ldots + \Sigma X_k^2 - (\Sigma X_k)^2/n$$

but is more simply found by difference.)

(v) Prepare the table:

Sources of variation	Sums-of-squares	Degrees of freedom	Mean-squares	F
Treatments	SST	$k-1$	$MST = SST/k-1$	MST/MSE
Error	SSE	$k(n-1)$	$MSE = SSE/k(n-1)$	—
(Total)	(SS)	$(kn-1)$	—	—

(vi) Enter the computed value of F in the table at $(k-1)$ numerator and $k(n-1)$ denominator degrees of freedom. If the computed value is equal to or exceeds the tabulated value for $P = 0.05$ we normally reject the null hypothesis and conclude that the samples represent populations with different means, in other words, there are significant differences between treatment means.*

NB Although experiments are usually planned with equal numbers of replicates per treatment we often need to apply analysis of variance when the numbers are not equal. Minor modifications in computation accommodate this. C becomes $(GT)^2/\Sigma n$, and SST becomes $\Sigma(T^2/n) - C$. The number of degrees of freedom for error becomes $\Sigma(n-1)$ or $\Sigma n - k$.

9.3 Comparisons between sample means

The analysis may be continued in either of two ways:

(i) *Partition of treatment sum-of-squares.* The treatment sum-of-squares, SST, with $(k-1)$ degrees of freedom has been extracted. For an analysis with only two treatments there is only one degree of freedom and the F test becomes equivalent to the corresponding t test. (Note that F, with numerator degrees of freedom = 1, is equal to t^2 with the same denominator degrees of freedom.) Many workers never use the t test,

---

* In this test we are interested only in values of $F > 1.0$ so the test is 'one-tailed'. The usual tables of F are labelled accordingly.

prefering to employ the analysis of variance technique irrespective of the number of treatments.

When the number of treatments exceeds two the treatment sum-of-squares may be partitioned to permit the testing of a number of different comparisons. If the logic of the situation requires it a whole series of comparisons, each with one degree of freedom, can be made. The sum-of-squares for a particular comparison may be computed as $\Sigma(T^2/n) - (\Sigma T)^2/\Sigma n$. When all treatments are included in the comparison $(\Sigma T)^2/\Sigma n = C$. Where T is now the sum of the values for one or more treatments included in a particular category for comparison and n is the total number of such values. Partition of treatment sum-of-squares may be justified even when preliminary analysis has failed to show significant overall variation between treatment means. The comparisons must be defined so that they are independent of one another. No attempt will be made here to explain this technique in detail but simple worked examples will be found in the solutions to Problems 9–3 and 9–4.

(ii) *Testing the significance of individual differences between treatment means.* Several methods are available for examining individual differences between treatment means but they should not be used indiscriminately. It is important to understand the problems involved in making multiple tests of significance so that experiments may be properly designed and appropriate methods of analysis selected. The following tests are normally only applied when the preliminary analysis of variance has indicated that there are significant differences between treatment means.

Least significant difference – L.S.D.

We have seen (§ 9.1) that if we make a long series of significance tests, each at the 5% level, we run a serious risk of making a Type 1 error. We can often reduce the severity of this problem by defining precisely the objects of our experiment or survey, deciding on the exact questions to which we require answers and *nominating in advance* the limited number of comparisons that we intend to make. We may then feel justified in making several such *a priori* comparisons at the usual 5% level of significance per test. To do this we can use, either the modified **t** test or the method of least significant difference.

When applying a **t** test we compute the ratio (difference)/(S.E. of difference). The true variances of the populations are assumed to be equal and the S.E. used in the test is computed from the combined data. In the mean-square for error in the analysis of variance we have an estimate of the error variance based on the combined data for all samples. The S.E. of the difference between two means of n then becomes $\sqrt{(2s^2/n)}$ where s^2 is the error mean-square. When $n_1 \neq n_2$ this takes the form $\sqrt{(s^2/n_1 + s^2/n_2)}$. This estimate may be used when making a comparison nominated *a priori*. The number of degrees of freedom for the test is $k(n-1)$ or $\Sigma n - k$ respectively. For a two-treatment analysis this will give a result identical to that of the usual t test but where there are more than two treatments it will tend to be more sensitive because of the larger number of degrees of freedom. NB s^2 may also be used to fit confidence limits to individual means (see § 2.5) and to differences between selected pairs of means (see (§ 3.2.).

Instead of evaluating t for a particular pair of means we can calculate the least difference between a pair of means (taken at random) which would be significant, as L.S.D. $= t_{0.05} \sqrt{(2s^2/n)}$, where t has $k(n-1)$ degrees of freedom. Pairs of means which differ by more than the L.S.D. may be regarded as significantly different. Such a test can only be applied when each sample contains an equal number of replicates. Having computed the L.S.D. it is very tempting to apply it to differences between all pairs of means, or pairs selected *a posteriori*. Such a temptation should be firmly resisted.

Fixed range test – using L.S.R.

Circumstances often arise in which we need to make a large number of comparisons between treatment means and/or to nominate comparisons *a posteriori*. We then need to modify the testing procedure to reduce the risk of making Type 1 errors. We can restate the expression for L.S.D. as $t_{0.05} \sqrt{2}(s/\sqrt{n})$ and see that the L.S.D. is the S.E. of an individual mean $\times t_{0.05} \sqrt{2}$. Assuming that all possible comparisons between treatment means will be made a multiplier $Q(\geqslant t \sqrt{2})$ has been devised which when used instead of $t \sqrt{2}$ reduces the probability of a Type 1 error *per analysis* to the probability level of Q employed, e.g. 0.05. We read Q from the table of the 'Studentized Range' (Table V) for the number of treatments in the analysis and for the number of degrees of freedom for error, i.e. $k(n-1)$.

Multiple range test – using S.S.R.

Use of the L.S.R. can substantially reduce the sensitivity of an experiment i.e. greatly increase the probability of making Type 2 errors. Several methods have been devised which while providing reasonable protection against Type 1 errors allow the retention of greater sensitivity. In these the means are arranged in order of magnitude and a series of shortest significant ranges, S.S.R.'s, is calculated for testing differences between pairs of means according to their relationship in the size order. As in the fixed-range test we first compute the S.E. of a treatment mean, i.e. $\sqrt{(s^2/n)}$. We then look up values of Q for the number of degrees of freedom for error and for $k, (k-1), (k-2), (k-3), \ldots 2$ treatments. We then compute the S.S.R.'s for groups of $k, (k-1), (k-2), (k-3) \ldots 2$, as $Q \sqrt{(s^2/n)}$. Having arranged the treatment means in order of magnitude we test the difference between the largest and smallest against the S.S.R. for k treatments. If this is non-significant we stop testing but if it is significant we test the differences between the largest and the next-to-smallest and the next-to-largest and the smallest against the SSR for $(k-1)$ treatments. We continue in this way for as long as differences prove significant but if a difference proves to be non-significant we do not test any differences within it. (See Problem 9–1.)

9.4 Assumptions underlying the analysis: transformation of data

Before considering further applications of the analysis of variance technique it is desirable to stop and consider the assumptions on which it is based so that it may be correctly applied. The two most important assumptions are:

(i) that the effects are additive, i.e. an individual value (of X) is considered to be made up of the grand mean + treatment effect* + uncontrolled error.

(ii) that the error is normally distributed and has equal variance for all treatments.

Fortunately these assumptions are satisfied for many biological data and so conclusions drawn from the analyses are valid. Not uncommonly, however, these assumptions are not justified and adjustments are required. A valuable form of adjustment is transformation of the original data (measurements, counts, %'s, etc.) by means of some mathematical function before analysis.

(i) Results in the form of small, whole-numbered counts tend to have a variance proportional to their mean (or equal to it, §5.2.). An appropriate transformation to render the variances independent of the means is $\sqrt{X}$ or when counts are low and zeros occur $\sqrt{(X + 0.5)}$.

(ii) Correlations between means and variances are not confined to counts and more generally the $\log X$ transformation, or $\log(X + 1)$ if zeros are present, is employed. The log transformation is also appropriate when responses tend to be proportional rather than additive, e.g. for treatments at levels 0, 1, 2, 4 yielding treatment means of 0, 10, 20, and 40, rather than 10, 12, 14, and 18.

(iii) Data in the form of probabilities, proportions or percentages tend to be binomially distributed (Chapter 4) but when the corresponding values of P range only from 0.0 to 0.2 a Poisson distribution is approached and $a\sqrt{X}$ or $\sqrt{(X + 0.5)}$ transformation is applicable. Values of p of 0.8 to 1.0 are subtracted from 1.0 and then treated similarly. When the range of p is 0.5 ± 0.2 the distribution is almost normal and transformation is likely to be unnecessary but where the range of p is greater the 'angular' or $\sin^{-1}\sqrt{p}$ transformation is called for.

* This is so for the 'Model 1' form of the analysis. For the 'Model 2' form see section 9.5.

Although arguments for data transformation are statistical it is often of value to enquire why the data need transformation. To do so may indicate how the data may have been collected so as not to require it, and even to throw some light on the phenomena which give rise to them. For example, it has been found that areas of fungal colonies require transformation but that the radii do not. This suggests that the important variable here is the distance of spread from the point of inoculation or infection. Similarly, total weights of plants and animals often prove unsatisfactory variates. The fact that log weight proves satisfactory suggests that the quantity which is responding to treatment is growth rate.

The need for transformation may be predicted from the form of the data (e.g. counts, percentages, etc.) or from a comparison between the sample variances. A simple significance test for differences between sample variances is the F_{max} test. The ratio of the largest variance in the set to the smallest is calculated and compared with the tabulated value of F_{max} (Table VI) for the number of treatments in the set and $(n-1)$ degrees of freedom, where n is the number of replicates per sample. (A more comprehensive test which provides for differing numbers of replicates is described in SNEDECOR and COCHRAN (1967), section 10.21 and ROHLF and SOKAL (1969), Box 13.1.) Where there are only two treatments the ratio of the larger over the smaller variance may be compared with the tabulated value of F at the appropriate numbers of degrees of freedom. This is a two-tailed test so the probability values of the usual F tables must be doubled. (See § 3.3. and Problem 9-1.)

9.5   Experimental design and efficiency

We have so far been learning how to deal with numerical data gathered from experiments or surveys without paying much attention to the design of the experiments and surveys themselves. This could be misleading because plans for collecting data and analysing them should be made at the same time, as two complementary parts of a single operation of testing a hypothesis (see § 1.1). This point is perhaps best understood by examining the relationship between experimental design and analysis of variance.

The simplest kind of experiment that we can imagine is one in which we keep constant all factors other than the one to be varied experimentally. Many physical and chemical experiments approximate to this ideal but in biology variation in material, handling, and environment occurs and leads to variation in the results that must be accepted as error. There are *three* essentials in dealing with such a situation.

(i) *Reduce error to a minimum.* We can keep individual errors to a minimum by such means as using uniform experimental material, precision in the application of treatments, and closely controlled environments. Sample errors may be reduced by increasing the number of replicates and increasing the size of counts.

(ii) *Avoid bias* (i.e. association of a particular kind of error with a particular treatment). We can avoid bias by the use of *randomization*, i.e. by assigning individuals to treatments by a method which gives each individual an equal chance of being assigned to each treatment. This is usually done with the aid of random numbers.

(iii) *Arrange to be able to distinguish variation due to error from variation due to treatments.* We have seen how we can use the technique of analysis of variance to separate the effects of treatments from the error and how we can use the ratio of the two corresponding mean-squares to test the significance of the former. The experimental design corresponding to this kind of analysis is the *fully randomized* design. Some rather more complex designs will be considered in Chapter 10.

We have considered the application of analysis of variance in a situation where the classes into which the individuals fall correspond to treatments for which we suppose there are fixed effects. This is the 'Model 1' form. The analysis may also be applied in a rather different situation, in which the classes correspond to random samples from a variable population. This is the 'Model 2' form. In such situations we are usually not interested in fitting confidence limits to sample means or in testing differences between them but only in estimating the variability of the samples and perhaps comparing this with the variability of the individuals in the samples. For an example of this kind of application see Problem 9–2.

9.6 Analysis of variance in regression

9.6.1 *Testing the significance of regression: single values of Y*

We have seen (section 8.6) that the significance of regression may be tested using t to test the deviation of b, the regression coefficient, from zero. Alternatively the test may be made by using F in an analysis of variance. We partition the total sum-of-squares of $Y(\Sigma y^2)$ into its two components, as before, divide each by its number of degrees of freedom to obtain mean-squares and compute F as Regression MS/Residual MS, thus:

Sources of variation	Sums-of-squares	Degrees of freedom	Mean-squares	F
Regression	$\dfrac{(\Sigma xy)^2}{\Sigma x^2}$	1	$\dfrac{\text{Regression SS}}{1}$	$\dfrac{\text{Regression MS}}{\text{Residual MS}}$
Residual	$\Sigma y^2 - \dfrac{(\Sigma xy)^2}{\Sigma x^2}$	$N-2$	$\dfrac{\text{Residual SS}}{(N-2)}$	—
(Total)	(Σy^2)	$(N-1)$	—	—

F has $1/(N-2)$ degrees of freedom. See Problem 9–5.

9.6.2 Testing the significance of regression: replicated values of Y

Experiments to investigate the relationship between a dependent variable and an independent one often employ several replicates at each level of the independent variable. The analysis of the resulting data requires a combination of regression analysis and analysis of variance. The sum-of-squares for between treatments (SST) has two components: one is the sum-of-squares accounted for by regression – the Regression SS, and the other is the sum-of-squares for the deviation of treatment means from the linear relationship – the Deviation SS. By partitioning SST in this way we can not only test the significance of the regression but also, by comparing the Deviation MS with the Error MS (i.e. MSE), test the significance of *deviations from* linearity. See Problem 9–6.

9.6.3. Comparison of 2 regression coefficients

Having computed regression equations for two independent sets of data we frequently need to compare the two regression coefficients. This again may be done by using a form of analysis of variance. The two residual mean squares are first compared (larger/smaller) by means of a 'two-tailed' F test. Only if the difference is non-significant is the comparison of regression coefficients likely to be valid. Using the data from the two regressions we compute three new sums-of-squares:

(i) The total sum-of-squares *not* accounted for by the two regressions, i.e. the sum of the two residual sums-of-squares.

(ii) The sum-of-squares which would remain *not* accounted for by a single regression line computed from pooled data. This is computed for summed values of Σx^2, Σxy, and Σy^2.

(iii) The sum-of-squares corresponding to the difference between the regression lines, i.e. (ii) − (i).

We test the significance of the difference by testing the mean-square from (iii) with one degree of freedom, over the mean-square from (i) with $(N_1 + N_2 - 4)$ degrees of freedom, in an F test. See Problem 9–7. (A more general method for comparing two or more regression coefficients is described in SOKAL and ROHLF (1969), section 14.9 and Box 18.4.)

Problems

9–1 In an experiment to investigate the effect of light quality on the rate of photosynthesis of *Anacystis* (a blue-green alga) six replicate cultures of the alga were irradiated with each of seven wavelength ranges of equal energy level. Net photosynthesis was estimated in terms of oxygen produced determined by the Winkler method. Results are given here as ml N/100 $Na_2S_2O_3$ solution.

Light quality	Replicates					
	1	2	3	4	5	6
Blue	5.50	5.00	6.20	5.50	5.00	6.60
Green	6.10	5.70	6.20	6.10	6.40	5.60
Yellow	15.70	16.60	16.80	17.10	17.40	16.60
Red	19.20	19.00	19.00	18.70	18.90	18.70
Far-red	4.70	3.90	4.35	4.40	3.53	3.75
Flourescent white	21.00	21.85	22.00	21.50	21.00	20.25
Incandescent white	21.10	22.00	21.50	22.00	20.20	21.30

Carry out preliminary analysis of variance and then group the treatment means using a multiple range test.

9–2 In an investigation of the effect of NaCN (sodium cyanide) on the uptake *in vitro* of a particular amino acid by intestinal preparations from a certain species of fish, it was found that each fish would give only about six preparations. Since it would be necessary to use more than one fish in each experiment a preliminary test was carried out to compare the variation between fish with the variation between preparations. Three preparations were made for each of four fish. The results, expressed as μ mol g^{-1} dry weight 20 min^{-1} period, were as follows:

Replicate	Fish			
	1	2	3	4
(i)	2.53	2.02	1.66	1.36
(ii)	2.04	1.92	1.92	1.15
(iii)	2.34	2.03	1.47	1.16

Analyse these data and report on the relationship between the variance due to differences between fish and that due to differences between replicate preparations from the same fish.

9–3 In an area of dune heath the vegetation consisted of a mosaic of *Calluna vulgaris* bushes, *Erica cinerea* bushes and a carpet of several pleurocarpous mosses. In order to examine the possible differential effect of plant cover on soil surface pH a transect was placed subjectively across the area and at every 10 cm the following observations were made:
(i) Plant cover type classified as $C = Calluna$; $E = Erica$, and $M =$ moss.

(ii) pH of a 1:2 suspension in water of a surface soil sample (top 1 cm). The results are summarized below:

	C	E	M	(Totals)
N	48	42	38	(128)
ΣX	281.91	243.24	213.85	(739.00)
ΣX^2	1657.5552	1410.4975	1205.4818	(4273.5345)

Carry out preliminary analysis of variance and, if significant, partition the SST to make appropriate comparisons between treatments.

9-4 During a study of the photoperiodic control of reproduction in the red alga *Porphyra*, an experiment was conducted to examine the effect of interrupting a long dark period with 30 min illumination by light of different wavelengths but equal energy levels. Ten replicates were used for each of five wavelength bands and the results were recorded in the form of sporangial counts for a standard volume of algal material. It was known that for data of this kind errors in sampling and counting tended to be proportional to number counted so logarithmic transformation was called for. Only red light was expected, on theoretical grounds, to have an effect, so it was decided *before the experiment was set up* that the mean for the red light treatment would be compared with that for each of the other treatments.

The results are summarized below:

Colour	Blue	Green	Yellow	Red	Far-red	(Total)
$\Sigma(\log X)$	38.846	38.905	38.429	36.037	38.657	(190.874)
$\Sigma(\log X)^2$	150.925	151.447	147.745	130.566	149.511	(730.194)

Complete the analysis of variance and compare the mean for red light with each of the other treatment means using (i) the method of L.S.D. and (ii) the method of L.S.R.

9-5 Test the significance of the regression for Problem 8-2 using the method of section 9.6.

9-6 The data for colony radius in Problem 8-2 were means of 6 replicates. The full data are given below:

Days from inoculation		3	5	7	9	11	13	15
	(1)	8	13	17	22	26	30	31
	(2)	8	13	18	24	27	30	31
Mean radius (mm)	(3)	7	13	17	22	26	29	30
	(4)	8	13	18	24	28	30	31
	(5)	7	13	18	24	27	30	31
	(6)	8	13	17	22	26	29	31

Analyse the data by the method in section 9.6. How are the conclusions affected?

9-7 In the experiment of Problem 8–2 the following results were obtained for media containing 10 and 20 mg 1^{-1} glucose.

Days from inoculation	3	5	7	9
10 mg 1^{-1}	5.7	9.0	12.0	16.0
20 mg 1^{-1}	6.5	11.2	16.0	19.8

Carry out regression analysis for these two glucose concentrations and compare the two regression coefficients (growth rates) by the method in section 9.6.

10 Analysis of Variance: Double Classification

10.1 Randomized-block design

We have considered briefly the essentials of experimental design and noted, on the one hand, the desirability of treating uniform experimental material under closely-controlled experimental conditions, and on the other hand, the need to employ adequate replication (§ 9.5). In practice these two aspects of experimental design are often found to conflict. With the scale of an investigation fixed by the number of treatments and the amount of replication needed to provide the required sensitivity it is often necessary to tolerate one or more forms of unwanted variation in experimental material, experimental conditions, timing, or even in the identity of the recorder. This kind of difficulty may often be overcome by the use of the *randomized-block* design. In this we define a number of 'blocks'* each of which includes at least one replicate for every treatment. We then concentrate our resources on establishing and maintaining *uniformity within blocks*. Uncontrolled *variation between blocks* is relatively unimportant because in the numerical analysis the resulting variation can be distinguished from both variation due to treatments and the error variation.

In biology there are many sources of variation which can be dealt with in this way, sources of variation which can be anticipated but not eliminated. Variation in experimental material can often be largely removed from error by forming blocks of organisms of similar age, size, genetic constitution or environmental history (cf. paired sample test, §3.5). Again, the effects of uncontrolled variation in environmental conditions may be reduced by treating as blocks individual greenhouse benches, incubators, etc. Once, for any reason, blocks have been defined it is desirable to associate with them as many other sources of unwanted variation as possible, e.g. whole blocks should be recorded at the same time and by the same observer. Where, of necessity, individual experiments are on a very small scale, replicate experiments may usefully be treated as blocks, the analysis providing not only a test of significance between treatment means but also a test of homogeneity between experiments (cf. § 7.5).

*Use of this term originates in agricultural field experimentation where 'blocks' were literally blocks of experimental plots.

10.2   Double classification: without replication

Consider the results of an experiment with k treatments, b blocks and one replicate per treatment per block. The data would have the form:

Blocks	Treatments					Block totals
	1	2	3	...	k	
1	X_{11}	X_{21}	X_{31}	...	X_{k1}	B_1
2	X_{12}	X_{22}	X_{32}	...	X_{k2}	B_2
			to			
b	X_{1b}	X_{2b}	X_{3b}	...	X_{kb}	B_b
Treatment totals	T_1	T_2	T_3	...	T_k	GT Grand total
Treatment means	$\overline{X}_1$	$\overline{X}_2$	$\overline{X}_3$	...	$\overline{X}_k$	$\overline{X}$ Grand mean

(i)   Compute $C = (GT)^2/kb$ (there are kb values of X)

(ii) Compute $SS = \Sigma X^2 - C$ (as § 9.2)

(iii) Compute $SST = \Sigma T^2/b - C$ (there are b values of X for each treatment)

(iv) Compute $SSB = \Sigma B^2/k - C$ (there are k values of X for each block)

(v)   Compute $SSE = SS - (SST + SSB)$

(vi) Prepare the table:

Sources of variation	Sums-of-squares	Degrees of freedom	Mean-squares	F
Treatments	SST	$k-1$	$MST = SST/k-1$	MST/MSE
Blocks	SSB	$b-1$	$MSB = SSB/b-1$	MSB/MSE
Error	SSE	$(k-1)(b-1)$	$MSE = SSE/(k-1)(b-1)$	—
(Total)	(SS)	$(kb-1)$	—	—

(vii) Compute F for treatments as mean-square for treatments over mean-square for error and enter it into the table at $k-1/(k-1)(b-1)$ degrees of freedom. Differences between treatment means may be analysed further using the methods in section 9.3. Compute F for blocks as mean-square for blocks over mean-square for error and enter it into the table at $b-1/(k-1)(b-1)$ degrees of freedom. If variation between blocks is significant the existence of heterogeneity is confirmed and use of the randomized-block design justified. If variation between blocks is not significant and especially if F for blocks is less than unity the value of the randomized-block design may be questioned and in any further experiments the fully-randomized design substituted.

10.3 Double classification: with replication

Where resources permit it is usually desirable to replicate treatments within blocks. Apart from increasing the total number of replicates and hence the sensitivity of the experiment this has the advantage of permitting the detection of interaction. The effects of treatments and the differences associated with blocks may be simply additive so that an individual value (of X) is made up of the grand mean + a treatment effect + a block effect + error. In other words: treatments have the same effect in all blocks and differences associated with blocks affect the results for all treatments equally. It very often happens, however, that effects are not simply additive. Responses to treatments differ among blocks and differences associated with blocks are not the same for all treatments. Such departure from the additive pattern is called interaction. With only one replicate per treatment per block we cannot separate interaction from error. In section 10.2 where a direct estimate of error is not possible the SSE as computed includes any interaction. (In using the corresponding error mean-square to test the mean-square for blocks we are assuming that there is no interaction!)

Consider the results of an experiment with k treatments, b blocks and n replicates per treatment per block. The data would have the form:

Blocks	Treatments					Block totals
	1	2	3	$\ldots$	k	
1	X_{111} to Q_{11} X_{11n}	X_{211} to Q_{21} X_{21n}	X_{311} to Q_{31} X_{31n}	$\ldots$	X_{k11} to Q_{k1} X_{k1n}	B_1
2	X_{121} to Q_{12} X_{12n}	X_{221} to Q_{22} X_{22n}	X_{321} to Q_{32} X_{32n}	$\ldots$	X_{k21} to Q_{k2} X_{k2n}	B_2
			$\ldots\ldots$ to $\ldots\ldots$			
b	X_{1b1} to Q_{1b} X_{1bn}	X_{2b1} to Q_{2b} X_{2bn}	X_{3b1} to Q_{3b} X_{3bn}	$\ldots$	X_{kb1} to Q_{kb} X_{kbn}	B_b
Treatment totals	T_1	T_2	T_3	$\ldots$	T_k	GT Grand total
Treatment means	$\bar{X}_1$	$\bar{X}_2$	$\bar{X}_3$	$\ldots$	$\bar{X}_k$	$\bar{X}$ Grand mean

(i)   Compute $C = GT^2/kbn$ (there are now kbn values of X)

(ii)   Compute $SS = \Sigma X^2 - C$ (as before)

(iii)   Compute $SSQ = \Sigma Q^2/n - C$ (there are now n replicates in each sub-class)

(iv)   Compute $SSE = SS - SSQ$ (error is now estimated from variation within sub-classes)

(v)   Compute $SST = \Sigma T^2/bn - C$ (there are now bn values for each treatment)

(vi)   Compute $SSB = \Sigma B^2/kn - C$ (there are now kn values in each block)

(vii)   Compute $SSTB = SSQ - (SST + SSB)$ (cf. estimate of error in § 10.2)

(viii)   Prepare the table:

Sources of variation	Sums-of squares	Degrees of freedom	Mean-squares	F
Treatments	SST	$(k-1)$	$MST = SST/(k-1)$	MST/MSI
Blocks	SSB	$(b-1)$	$MSB = SSB/(b-1)$	MSB/MSE
Interaction	SSTB	$(k-1)(b-1)$	$MSI = SSTB/(k-1)(b-1)$	MSI/MSE
Error	SSE	$kb(n-1)$	$MSE = SSE/kb(n-1)$	—
(Total)	(SS)	$(kbn-1)$	—	—

(ix) Compute F for interaction as mean-square for interaction over mean-square for error and enter it into the table at $(k-1)(b-1)/kb(n-1)$ degrees of freedom.

(a) If interaction is significant (i.e. $P \leqslant 0.05$) differences between treatments vary from block to block and overall statements about treatment effects may not be possible. Draw up a table of sub-class totals (Q's) or sub-class means (Q/n's) and study for meaning. Alternatively display these values graphically. If interaction is very strong the assumptions on which the experiment was based should be reconsidered. It is sometimes useful to regard the experiment as several small experiments, one for each block, and to reanalyse each by the methods of Chapter 9. It may be desirable to investigate the causes of the interaction or, at least, to modify the design of further experiments. If the interaction is weak compared with the treatment effects complete the significance testing by computing F for blocks as mean-square for blocks over mean-square for error and enter the table at $(b-1)/kb(n-1)$ degrees of freedom. The interpretation of this is as for section 10.2. Compute F for treatments as mean-square for treatments over *mean-square for interaction* and enter the table at $(k-1)/(k-1)(b-1)$ degrees of freedom. Differences between treatment means may be analysed further employing the methods in section 9.3 but using the *interaction mean-square* as the estimate of error, with $(k-1)(b-1)$ degrees of freedom.

(b) If interaction is not significant (i.e. $P > 0.05$) we can retain the hypothesis of additivity on which the randomized-block design is based and continue with significance testing. The significance of variation between blocks may be tested by computing F for blocks as MSB/MSE as in (a) above. The interpretation of the result of this test is the same as for section 10.2 and (a) above. The significance of differences between treatments may be tested by computing F for treatments as MST/MSI as in (a) above. Differences between treatment means may be analysed further employing the methods of section 9.3 but using MSI as the estimate of error.

(c) If F for interaction is less than unity it may be safe to conclude that interaction is absent. In such a case both MSI and MSE are estimates of error alone and an improved estimate of error may be made by pooling the data. Again enter F for interaction into the table and compare it with the tabulated value for $P = 0.75$* at the appropriate numbers of degrees of freedom. If the computed value is *less* than the tabulated value (i.e. if interaction is not significant at $P = 0.75$) a pooled estimate of error may be made based on a greater number of degrees of freedom. To do this compute: $\text{MSE}_{pooled} = (\text{SSTB} + \text{SSE})/[(k-1)(b-1) + kb(n-1)]$. This new estimate may now be used to compute a revised value for F for treatments and in making comparisons between treatments when employing the methods in section 9.3.

10.4   Other double-classification designs

The analysis of variance with double-classification has so far been considered only in the context of making comparisons between treatment means. In the fully-randomized design (see § 9.2 and 9.3) we compare variation due to treatments with that for replicates within treatments. The randomized-block design can increase the sensitivity and hence the efficiency of experiments by associating in blocks sources of error that can be anticipated but not eliminated. The resulting variation can be separated from that due to treatments on the one hand and that between replicates on the other. If interaction is demonstrated the initial hypothesis of additivity must be rejected and allowances made when making inclusive statements, e.g. statements about treatments which are to apply to all blocks. Interaction is not always unexpected and unwanted. In some fields of enquiry the investigation of interaction is an important part of the work. Interactions between the different nutrient elements applied in plant nutrition experiments may be as important as the responses to the individual elements. In their simplest form such experiments require very little modification in the form of analysis. Several categories of one variable are treated as treatments and several

---

*   e.g. Table 5 of ROHLF and SOKAL (1969).

categories of the other as blocks. Analysis may yield conclusions relating to both main effects and to their interaction.

We have noted already in section 9.5 the difference between 'Model 1' and 'Model 2' in relation to single-classification designs. The randomized-block design is a Mixed Model, the treatment effects are fixed, i.e. 'Model 1', and the differences between blocks are random, i.e. 'Model 2'. (This is why MST and MSB are tested over different MS's in section 10.3.) The corresponding $k_1 \times k_2$ design with two sets of treatments is wholly 'Model 1'. The analysis is carried out as described in section 10.3 but significance testing takes a rather different course. Both mean-squares for treatments (one replacing MSB) and the mean-square for interaction are tested over the *mean-square for error*. In the absence of significant interaction the error mean-square may be used in the further analysis of the effects of both sets of treatments. A pooled estimate of error may be made if the conditions in section 10.3 (ix)(c) are satisfied.

Double classification designs can occur in which both classifications yield classes corresponding to random samples from variable populations. Such designs are wholly 'Model 2'. Analysis is carried out as described in section 10.3 but the mean-squares for both classifications are tested over the *mean-square for interaction*. The mean-square for interaction is tested over the mean-square for error in the usual way. Detailed comparisons between treatment means are not usually required.

10.5   Nested designs

There are other designs which involve double or even multiple classification but in which the classifications are not independent (as in § 10.2 to 10.4) but hierarchal. In many investigations populations are represented by samples consisting of a series of independent individuals of equal status, each contributing a single measurement, count, percentage, etc. Not infrequently however individuals contribute a number of measurements, and thus become sub-samples. The sub-samples themselves may consist of several sub-sub-samples each contributing several measurements. For example, where an experimental population consists of whole organisms each organism in a sample may be represented by several tissue preparations and each preparation by several determinations. The resulting nested designs can vary greatly in efficiency so it is important not only to be able to analyse the data from them correctly but also to appreciate the relative value of replication at the several levels.

A student proposed to investigate the effect of different light intensities on the mean chloroplast number per cell in the leaves of the moss *Funaria hygrometrica*. Decisions were needed on the number of cells to be counted per leaf, the number of leaves to be examined per sample and the number of samples to be examined per light intensity. To facilitate these decisions a trial was carried out in which the chloroplasts in each of ten cells, in each of five leaves, for each of four plant samples taken from a single light intensity, were counted. The results were as follows:

Sample		Leaf						
		1	2	3	4	5		(Totals)
1	ΣX	134	126	127	135	132	(654)	
	ΣX^2	1814	1622	1625	1867	1792		(8720)
2	ΣX	145	130	148	139	140	(702)	
	ΣX^2	2141	1712	2198	2039	1992		(10082)
3	ΣX	146	147	143	152	149	(737)	
	ΣX^2	2174	2167	2079	2314	2239		(10973)
4	ΣX	140	121	134	146	145	(686)	
	ΣX^2	1980	1495	1818	2132	2188		(9613)
							(2779)	(39388)

We need to divide the total sum-of-squares into three components, (i) between samples, (ii) between leaves within samples, and (iii) between counts within leaves.

$C = 2779^2/200 = 38\,614.21$

SS counts $= 39\,388 - C = 773.79$

SS leaves $= (134^2 + 126^2 + 127^2 + \ldots + 145^2)/10 - C = 143.49$

SS samples $= (654^2 + 702^2 + 737^2 + 686^2)/50 - C = 71.49$

Then by subtraction:

SS between leaves within samples $= 143.49 - 71.49 = 72.00$

SS between counts within leaves $= 773.79 - 143.49 = 630.30$

Sources of variation	Sums-of-squares	Degrees of freedom	Mean-squares	F
Samples	71.49	3	23.83	5.30**
Leaves within samples	72.00	16	4.50	1.29 NS
Counts within leaves	630.30	180	3.50	—
(Total)	(773.79)	(199)	—	—

The number of degrees of freedom for examining variation between the four samples is $(4 - 1) = 3$. The total number of degrees of freedom between 20 leaves is $(20 - 1) = 19$, but three of these are already being used for between-sample comparisons, leaving $(19-3) = 16$ for *between leaves within samples*. A similar argument applies to the number of degrees of freedom for counts within leaves, i.e. $(199 - 19) = 180$. In this kind of analysis the mean-square at any level estimates the variance at that level plus those for all lower levels. Tests of significance are therefore normally made by comparing the mean square at a particular level over the next below it.

F for between leaves within samples $4.30/3.50 = 1.29$, with $16/180$ degrees of freedom gives $P > 0.1$. F for between samples $23.83/4.50 = 5.30$ with $3/16$ degrees of freedom gives $P < 0.01$. The trial then indicates that there is a highly-significant added variance component between samples and that greater efficiency in estimating mean chloroplast number per cell for a particular light intensity would be obtained by using a larger number of plant samples and counting chloroplasts in a smaller number of cells in fewer leaves of each. In practice the decisions on the amount of replication at each level would take into account the availability of plant material and the relative times involved.

The design of the trial above is entirely 'Model 2'. The design of the full investigation, including the comparison of light intensities would be a Mixed Model with the first level (light intensities) being 'Model 1'. In such a design, if F for the second level (samples) is less than unity, pooling to increase the number of degrees of freedom for 'within samples' may be carried out if the conditions in section 10.3, (ix) (c) are satisfied. (See Problem 10.5.)

Problems

10–1 The experiment described in Problem 9–1 was a class experiment in which each column in the table was the responsibility of an individual student. Extend the analysis of the data to test for errors associated with students by treating students as blocks. How are the conclusions affected?

10–2 Because of the relatively large variation between fish revealed by the preliminary test of Problem 9–2, a two-treatment experiment, with and without NaCN, was carried out using a randomized-block design and with four fish as blocks.

	Fish			
	1	2	3	4
Without NaCN	1.54	1.52	1.00	1.58
	1.92	2.02	1.12	1.78
	2.26	1.91	1.13	1.52
With NaCN	1.10	1.31	0.79	1.24
	1.42	1.15	0.84	0.81
	1.04	1.51	0.86	1.32

Analyse the data by the method in 10.3. State, with 95% confidence limits, the effect of adding NaCN to the medium.

10–3   As part of an investigation into factors controlling the morphogenesis of fern gametophytes a 2×2 factorial experiment was set up in which suspensions of fern spores in nutrient medium were treated as follows:
(i) Control = nutrient medium only.
(ii) + 80 ppm (v/v) ethanol
(iii) + 20 ppm (v/v) acetaldehyde (ethanal)
(iv) + 80 ppm (v/v) ethanol + 20 ppm (v/v) acetaldehyde
Thirty days after sowing 20 gametophytes from each treatment were taken at random and their lengths measured in arbitrary micrometer units. The results were as follows:

			$-$ Ethanol	$+$
Acetaldehyde	$-$	ΣX	2255	2994
		ΣX^2	269 159	453 356
	$+$	ΣX	731	1233
		ΣX^2	30 269	77 543

Complete the analysis of variance and state the effects of 80 ppm ethanol and 20 ppm acetaldehyde on the development of fern gametophytes.

10–4   At the same time as the lengths of the gametophytes referred to in Problem 10–3 were measured their total cell number was also recorded. The results, after transformation to $\sqrt{X}$, were as follows:

		−	*Ethanol*	+
Acetaldehyde	−	ΣX	76.281	62.014
		ΣX^2	295	197
	+	ΣX	38.034	47.992
		ΣX^2	76	119

Complete the analysis of variance as you see fit. What conclusions do you draw?

10–5 Three groups of 12 litters each of three gerbils (*Meriones unguiculatus*) were reared under each of the following three social conditions.

A Male present: female pregnant
B Male absent from day 2: female pregnant
C Male absent from day 0: female *not* pregnant
The offspring were weighed at 25 days.
Results: (weights in grams)

						Litter						
	1	2	3	4	5	6	7	8	9	10	11	12
A	24.7	24.3	19.8	22.1	17.5	19.1	16.3	18.3	15.8	22.5	20.4	20.6
	24.2	23.3	19.2	21.9	19.3	20.3	16.8	17.5	15.1	25.3	19.4	21.5
	24.3	23.7	18.7	21.3	17.8	20.3	17.7	19.3	17.0	23.0	21.8	20.8
B	20.2	17.8	19.8	15.1	16.6	20.5	20.7	19.7	17.0	22.8	17.5	18.6
	20.9	15.3	22.0	13.8	17.5	20.2	20.3	18.7	16.4	23.8	16.4	17.3
	20.1	18.3	19.3	13.5	17.0	20.7	19.4	21.4	13.8	23.9	18.1	19.6
C	16.8	23.7	22.0	20.5	22.2	20.0	18.3	18.0	20.4	17.5	24.0	19.0
	17.4	21.6	22.0	19.7	22.9	19.6	18.4	17.2	18.6	15.2	24.3	17.2
	17.4	23.1	20.7	19.5	21.6	21.9	18.5	17.0	20.5	16.1	25.8	18.9

Analyse these data using the method in section 10.5. Then re-analyse the data *incorrectly* ignoring the classification into litters, i.e. using the method in section 9.2. What are the differences in the conclusions reached?

10–6 In the data of Problem 9–6 each row corresponds to an individual colony which was measured at 2-day intervals. Extend the analysis by treating the colonies as blocks.

Solutions to Problems

Chapter 1

1-1   Five beetles. For a significant departure from expectation an outcome must have a probability of $\leqslant 0.05$. Assuming $p = 0.5$ the probability of all beetles in a group moving to high humidity is $0.5^5 = 0.031\,25\,(1/32)$ which is < 0.05. The corresponding probability for a group of four beetles would be $0.5^4 = 0.0625\,(1/16)$ which is > 0.05.

1-2   As the family may be all boys or all girls the test is 'two-tailed'. The probability of a family of six children all the same sex is $2(0.5)^6 = 0.031\,25$. This is the smallest family to correspond to a probability of < 0.05 and therefore to lead to rejection of the hypothesis. It should be remembered that the selection of 0.05 as the critical level for statistical significance, although conventional, is quite arbitrary.

    A biologist with a family of six girls could still rationally welcome a seventh child in the hope that it would be a boy.

Chapter 2

2-1 $N = 12;\ \Sigma X = 624.4;\ \bar{X} = 52.03;\ \Sigma X^2 = 33\,244.78$

$$\text{S.E. of mean} = \sqrt{\left(\dfrac{33\,244.78 - \dfrac{624.4^2}{12}}{11 \times 12}\right)} = 2.392$$

    95% confidence limits $52.03 \pm 2.201 \times 2.392$
               i.e. $52.03 \pm 5.26\ (46.77 \text{ to } 57.29)$

2-2   The 95% confidence limits are $\bar{X} \pm 2.064 \times s/\sqrt{25}$. If the total number of replicates to give the required 99% limits is N then the 99% limits are (approx) $\bar{X} \pm 2.797 \times s/\sqrt{N}$. So, placing $2.064/\sqrt{25} = 2.797/\sqrt{N}$ gives $N = 46$ (to nearest integer). Since 25 determinations have been made already 21 further determinations will probably be required.

2-3   The 95% limits are to be $\bar{X} \pm 1.0$ mm. So the S.E. of the mean will be (approx.) $1.0/1.96$. But the S.E. of the mean is also $s/\sqrt{N}$, where N is the number of replicates required. As $s = 5$, we can equate $5/\sqrt{N} = 1.0/1.96$, giving $N = 96$ (to nearest integer). The taxonomist should, therefore, take 60 more measurements.

2–4 Confidence limits are computed as $\overline{X} \pm t \times s/\sqrt{N}$, where N is the number of replicates, $s/\sqrt{N}$ is the estimated S.E. of the mean and t has $(N-1)$ degrees of freedom. Clearly, to halve $s/\sqrt{N}$ the value of N must be quadrupled, i.e. increased to 20. But this would also reduce the value of t, so:

In the trial $\quad \overline{X} \pm 2.776 \times s/\sqrt{5} = 1.241s$
With $N = 20$ $\quad \overline{X} \pm 2.093 \times s/\sqrt{20} = 0.468s$

So, assuming the two values of s to be equal this would reduce the confidence limits by 62%. Testing other values of N we find that $N = 13$ gives a reduction of 51.3% and $N = 12$ gives a reduction of 48.8%. These predictions are estimates only and may prove misleading if the value of s computed for the original five replicates proves later to deviate markedly from the population standard deviation (σ).

Chapter 3

3–1 $\quad s_c^2 = \dfrac{(121.52 - 109^2/100 + 83.60 - 80.8^2/80)}{178} = 0.026\,416$

$s_c = 0.1625$

$$t = \frac{0.080}{0.1625\sqrt{\left(\dfrac{1}{100} + \dfrac{1}{80}\right)}} = \frac{0.080}{0.024\,38} = \underline{3.281} \text{ with 178 degrees of freedom}$$

This value corresponds to a probability just greater than 0.001.

3–2

	Island J	Island K
ΣX	1611	2009
N	15	20
$\overline{X}$	107.40	100.45
ΣX^2	174\,027	202\,123
s^2	71.83	16.79

$t = \dfrac{107.40 - 100.45}{\sqrt{(71.83/15 + 16.79/20)}} = \dfrac{6.95}{2.372} = 2.930$

$u = \dfrac{71.83/15}{71.83/15 + 16.79/20} = \dfrac{4.789}{5.628} = 0.851$

$1/f = 0.0517 + 0.0012 \qquad\qquad = 0.0529$

$f = \underline{18.9}$, or to nearest integer 19 degrees of freedom.

The computed value of t (2.930) exceeds the tabulated value for $P = 0.01$ at 19 degrees of freedom.

3–3

	Before	*After*
ΣX	1182	1288
N	14	14
$\overline{X}$	84.43	92.00
ΣX^2	101 456	120 022

$$s_c^2 = \frac{(101\,456 - 1182^2/14 + 120\,022 - 1288^2/14)}{14 + 14 - 2} = 122.59$$

$$s_c = 11.07$$

$$t = \frac{7.57}{11.07\,\sqrt{(1/14 + 1/14)}} = \underline{1.81}, \text{ with 26 degrees of freedom, giving } P > 0.05$$

We conclude that the two mean pulse rates, before and after eating, are *not* significantly different.

3–4   Mean difference, $\overline{Z} = 637/50 = 12.74$ cm

S.E. of mean difference $= \sqrt{\left(\dfrac{14\,433 - 637^2/50}{50 \times 49}\right)} = 1.606$

$t = 12.74/1.606 = \underline{7.93}$, with 49 degrees of freedom, giving $P < 0.001$. We conclude that the *mean difference* is very highly significant but can draw no conclusion about the difference between the mean depth of the soil where *Nardus* is present and the mean depth where it is absent. (cf. worked example in section 3.4 and Problem 3–3.)

Chapter 4

4–1 $n = 50$, $X = 30$, $p = 30/50 = 0.6$, $q = 1 - 0.6 = 0.4$
hatchability percentage $= 100p = 60\%$

(a) S. E. of percentage $= \sqrt{(60 \times 40/50)} = 6.928$

95% limits (approx.) $60\% \pm 1.96 \times 6.928$
± 13.58, i.e. **46.42 to 73.58**%

(b) 95% limits of p

$$\frac{0.6 + 1.96^2/100 \pm 1.96/\sqrt{50}\,\sqrt{(0.6 \times 0.4 + 1.96^2/200)}}{1 + 1.96^2/50}$$

$= 0.4618$ to 0.7239, giving 95% limits of percentage **46.18 to 72.39**%

4–2 $n = 200$, $X = 50$, $p = 50/200 = 0.25$, $q = 1 - 0.25 = 0.75$
cover percentage $= 100 \times 0.25 = 25\%$
(a) S.E. of percentage $= \sqrt{(25 \times 75/200)} = 3.062$
    95% limits (approx.) $25\% \pm 1.96 \times 3.062$
    ± 6.00, i.e. 19.00 to 31.00%
(b) 95% limits of p

$$\frac{0.25 + 1.96^2/400 \pm 1.96/\sqrt{200}\,\sqrt{(0.25 \times 0.75 + 1.96^2/800)}}{1 + 1.96^2/200}$$

$= 0.1951$ to 0.3143, giving 95% limits of percentage 19.51
    to 31.43%
95% limits are $\pm 1.96\,\sqrt{(25 \times 75/N)}$ so for limits of $\pm 1\%$ equate
this expression to unity and solve for N, thus:
$N = 1.96^2 \times 25 \times 75 = 7203$, i.e. approx 7200 point quadrats

4–3 $n = 100$, $X = 100$, $p = 100/100 = 1.0$, $q = 1 - 1.0 = 0$
(a) S.E. of percentage $= \sqrt{(100 \times 0/100)} = 0$
    95% limits (approx.) 100 ± 0, i.e. 100 to 100%
(b) 95% limits of p

$$\frac{1 + 1.96^2/200 \pm 1.96/\sqrt{100}\,\sqrt{(1 \times 0 + 1.96^2/400)}}{1 + 1.96^2/100}$$

$= 0.963$ to 1.000, giving 95% limits of percentage 96.3 to
    100%

4–4   (a) Individual terms of $(0.5 + 0.5)^{20}$:

p_{20}	9.5367×10^{-7}
p_{19}	1.9073×10^{-5}
p_{18}	1.8120×10^{-4}
p_{17}	1.0872×10^{-3}
p_{16}	4.6206×10^{-3}
p_{15}	1.4786×10^{-2}
(Total)	(2.0695×10^{-2}) ('one tail')

Sum of 'two tails' (NB $p = 0.5 = q$) $= 4.139 \times 10^{-2}$
i.e. 0.0414, which is < 0.05

(b) $n = 20$, $p = 0.5$, $pn = 10$, $X = 15$

$$d = \frac{|15-10| - 0.5}{\sqrt{(0.5 \times 0.5 \times 20)}} = 2.0125, \text{ giving } P < 0.05$$

4–5   If the probability of all 10 seeds germinating is 0.5,
$p = \sqrt[10]{0.5} = 0.9330$, and percentage germination $= 93.30\%$

4–6 $p = 0.2$, $q = 0.8$, and $n = 6$
Probabilities of getting 6, 5, 4, 3, 2, 1 and 0 questions correct are given by $(0.2 + 0.8)^6$. To score 50% or more 3, 4, 5, or 6 questions must be answered correctly. Total probability: $0.0001 + 0.0015 + 0.0154 + 0.0819 = 0.0989$, which is rather less than $1:10$. The candidate has about a 10% chance of passing the paper by selecting answers at random.

4–7   Single seeds:
percentage germination
$$= \frac{344}{400} \times 100 = 86\%$$

Paired seeds:
$\Sigma X = 240$, $\Sigma X^2 = 404$

∴ Percentage germination
$$= \frac{240}{400} \times 100 = 60\%$$

Observed variance
$$= \frac{404 - 240^2/200}{199} = 0.5829$$

Expected variance $= 0.6 \times 0.4 \times 2 = 0.48$

S.E. of difference
$$= \sqrt{\left(\frac{2 \times 0.48^2}{199} + \frac{0.48(1 - 6 \times 0.4 \times 0.6)}{200} \right)}$$
$$= 0.035\,49$$

$t = \dfrac{0.5829 - 0.48}{0.035\,49}$ $= 2.900$, with 199 degrees of freedom, giving $P < 0.01$

$\chi^2 = 116/0.48$ $= 241.6$, with 199 degrees of freedom, giving $P < 0.01$

As the paired seeds do not behave independently we may not treat the 200 pairs as a single sample in a test of significance. Treat the data for both treatments as for 200 samples of two seeds and compare the mean numbers germinating *per sample* by means of a d test. For paired seeds use the observed variance computed above and for the single seeds use expected binomial variance, thus:

	Single	Paired
Mean number germinating per sample of 2	1.72	1.20
Variance of number germinating per sample	0.2408	0.5829

$$d = \frac{1.72 - 1.20}{\sqrt{\left(\dfrac{0.2408}{200} + \dfrac{0.5829}{200}\right)}} = 8.103, \text{ giving } P < 0.001$$

4–8 $\Sigma X = 320$, $\Sigma X^2 = 808$

percentage cover $= \dfrac{320 \times 100}{200 \times 5} = 32\%$

Observed variance $= \dfrac{808 - 320^2/200}{199} = 1.4874$

Expected variance $= 0.32 \times 0.68 \times 5 = 1.088$

S.E. of difference $= \sqrt{\left(2 \times 1.088^2 + \dfrac{1.088(1 - 6 \times 0.32 \times 0.68)}{200}\right)}$

$= 0.1012$

$t = \dfrac{1.4874 - 1.088}{0.1012} = 3.947$, with 199 degrees of freedom, giving $P < 0.001$

$\chi^2 = 296/1.088 = 272.06$, with 199 degrees of freedom, giving $P < 0.001$

The observed variance of the number of hits per group of five point-quadrats is highly-significantly greater that the expected variance. This indicates that the clover is distributed in dense patches, the patches probably approaching 0.4 m in diameter.

Chapter 5

5–1 Let the number to be counted be M then (using the approximate formula) 95% limits would be $\pm 1.96 \sqrt{M}$, but the limits are to be $\pm 5\%$ M, so we equate $1.96 \sqrt{M} = (5/100)M$. So: $1.96^2 M = M^2/400$ and $M = 400 \times 1.96^2 = 1536.64$, or approximately 1550 organisms.

5–2 Y has a rate of $165/5 = 33 \text{ min}^{-1}$
Z has a rate of $120/3 = 40 \text{ min}^{-1}$

$$d = \frac{|165 - (165 + 120)(5/(5 + 3))| - 0.5}{\sqrt{[(165 + 120)(5/(5 + 3))(3/(5 + 3))]}} = \frac{12.625}{8.173} = 1.545,$$

giving $P > 0.1$, so they are not significantly different.

5-3 $d = \dfrac{|317 - 285| - 0.5}{\sqrt{317}} = \dfrac{31.5}{17.8} = 1.769$

As a fall in background rate is not considered this is a one-tailed test and we halve the tabulated probability values. $d = 1.769$ gives $P < 0.05$ for a one-tailed test, so the increase in rate is significant at the 95% level.

5-4   By the method in section 2.4. $\Sigma X = 460$ and $\Sigma X^2 = 1742$
Mean density $= 460/200 = 2.30$
Observed variance $= (1742 - 460^2/200)/199 = 3.4372.$
Variance/mean $= 3.4372/2.30 = 1.4944$
S.E. of ratio $= \sqrt{(2/199)}\quad = 0.100\,25$

$t = \dfrac{1.4944 - 1}{0.10025} = 4.932$, with 199 degrees of freedom,
giving $P < 0.001$

Alternatively: $\chi^2 = 684/2.30 = 297.39$, with 199 degrees of freedom, giving $P < 0.001$

We conclude that the plants are not randomly distributed and as the variance/mean ratio is > 1.0 they are contagiously distributed, i.e. they tend to occur in high density patches.

5-5   The packets may be regarded as equal random samples of the weed seed population, with a mean of 1.5. We need the probability of from four to ∞ seeds occurring. Compute the sum of the first four terms of the corresponding Poisson distribution and subtract this from 1.0:

$e^{-1.5}$	0.223 13
$e^{-1.5} \times 1.5$	0.334 70
$e^{-1.5} \times 1.5^2/2!$	0.251 02
$e^{-1.5} \times 1.5^3/3!$	0.125 51
(Total)	(0.934 36)

$1.0 - 0.934\,36 = 0.065\,36 = 0.065\,64$, which is approximately $1:15$

Chapter 6

6-1

Class	Observed frequency	Expected frequency	Deviation
Red-eyed	768	793	−25
White-eyed	818	793	+25
(Total)	(1586)	(1586)	(00)

$$\chi^2 = \frac{(-24.5)^2}{793} + \frac{24.5^2}{793} = 1.51, \text{ with one degree of freedom,}$$
$$\text{giving } P > 0.05$$

The deviation from expectation is therefore not significant.

6-2

Class	Observed frequency	Expected frequency	Deviation
Full-winged	2492	2367	+125
Vestigial-winged	664	789	−125
(Total)	(3156)	(3156)	(000)

$$\chi^2 = \frac{124.5^2}{2367} + \frac{(-124.5)^2}{789} = 26.2, \text{ with one degree of freedom,}$$
$$\text{giving } P < 0.001$$

The deviation from expectation is therefore very highly significant. The counts for the vestigial-winged flies were markedly below expectation for some bottles only. In these the food material had become unusually sticky and had trapped many of the relatively inactive vestigial-winged flies.

6-3 If the seeds in pairs behave independently the numbers germinated would approach the terms of the binomial expansion $200(0.6 + 0.4)^2$.

Number germinated	2	1	0
Observed frequency	82	76	42
Expected frequency	72	96	32

$$\chi^2 = \frac{10^2}{72} + \frac{(-20)^2}{96} + \frac{10^2}{32} = \underline{8.68}, \text{ with one degree of freedom,}$$
$$\text{giving } P < 0.01$$

This test thus again leads to the rejection of the hypothesis of independence (Problem 4–7). We note that the observed frequencies of '2-germinated' and '0-germinated' both exceed expectation suggesting some form of positive interaction. Any new hypothesis should take account of this and the lower germination percentage of the paired seeds.

6–4 If the points in the groups behave as independent point quadrats the numbers of hits recorded would approach the binomial expansion $200(0.32 + 0.68)^5$.

Number of hits	5	4	3	2	1	0
Observed frequency	4	13	26	48	74	35
Expected frequency	0.67	7.13	30.30	64.40	68.42	29.08

$$\chi^2 = \frac{9.2^2}{7.80} + \frac{(-4.3)^2}{30.30} + \frac{(-16.4)^2}{64.40} + \frac{5.58^2}{68.42} + \frac{5.92^2}{29.08} = \underline{17.30},$$

with three degrees of freedom, giving $P < 0.001$. This agrees with earlier tests.

6–5 If the plants are randomly distributed the frequencies of 0's, 1's, 2's, 3's, and etc would approach the terms of the Poisson expansion: $200e^{-2.3}(1, 2.3, \dfrac{2.3^2}{2!}, \dfrac{2.3^3}{3!}, \dfrac{2.3^4}{4!}, \text{etc.})$

No. of plants	0	1	2	3	4	5	6	7	8	9	10
Observed frequency	31	48	44	33	18	13	7	3	2	1	0
									(13)		
Expected frequency	20.05	46.12	53.04	40.66	23.38	10.76	4.12	1.35	0.39	0.10	0.02
									(5.98)		

$$\chi^2 = \frac{10.95^2}{20.05} + \frac{1.88^2}{46.12} + \frac{(-9.04)^2}{53.04} + \frac{(-7.66)^2}{40.66} + \frac{(-5.38)^2}{23.38}$$
$$+ \frac{2.24^2}{10.76} + \frac{7.02^2}{5.98}$$

$= \underline{18.99}$, with five degrees of freedom, giving $P < 0.01$
This agrees with earlier tests but at a lower level of significance.

This is probably due to some loss of sensitivity in the goodness-of-fit test as a result of pooling the terms with the lowest expected frequencies.

Chapter 7

7–1 Set up a 2×2 table, obtaining the remaining frequencies by subtraction, thus:

		Clover		
		+	−	
	+	90	25	(115)
Casts	−	170	115	(285)
		(260)	(140)	(400)

$$\chi^2 = \frac{400(90 \times 115 - 25 \times 170 - 200)^2}{115 \times 285 \times 260 \times 140}$$

$= \underline{11.67}$, with one degree of freedom, giving $P < 0.001$

Highly significant association is indicated and as (ad) exceeds (bc) the association is positive.

7–2 Set up a 6×2 table and calculate expected frequencies from the marginal totals, thus:

		< 30	30–39	40–49	50—59	60–69	⩾ 70	(Total)
A	O	3	8	32	18	12	5	(78)
	E	4.98	11.06	29.87	16.60	11.06	4.43	
B	O	6	12	22	12	8	3	(63)
	E	4.02	8.94	24.13	13.40	8.94	3.57	
	(Total)	(9)	(20)	(54)	(30)	(20)	(8)	(141)

Four expected frequencies are less than five, but since none approaches unity the analysis may be completed without pooling. (Alternatively, the observed frequencies for both < 30 and $\geqslant 70$ could be added to those of the adjacent columns to produce a 4×2 table.) Compute χ^2 as $\Sigma(O^2/E) - n$.

$\chi^2 = 1.81 + 5.79 + 34.28 + 19.52 + \ldots$ etc. $\ldots + 2.52 - 141$
$= \underline{4.62}$, with five degrees of freedom, giving P about 0.5.

We conclude that the results do not show significant heterogeneity.

7–3   We now have a 2×4 table, thus:

Batch	Wild type	Mutant	(Total)	χ^2 for overall segregation
1	60	26	(86)	$= \dfrac{(270-276)^2}{276} + \dfrac{(98-92)^2}{92} = 0.5222,$
2	75	33	(108)	
3	81	18	(99)	
5	54	21	(75)	
(Total)	(270)	(98)	(368)	with one degree of freedom.

Total χ^2 value (sum of individual χ^2 values for the four batches) $= 1.256 + 1.778 + 2.455 + 0.360 = \underline{5.849}$, with four degrees of freedom. Compute χ^2 for heterogeneity and display the results:

Sources of variation	Degrees of freedom	χ^2	Probability
Deviation from 3:1 ratio	1	0.522	> 0.1
Heterogeneity	3	5.327	> 0.1
(Total)	(4)	(5.849)	—

We conclude that the data are homogeneous and do not deviate significantly from the expected ratio of $3:1$.

7–4   Set up a 2×4 table and insert expected values, thus:

	Male	(Expected)	Female	(Total)
Control	34	(32.5)	31	(65)
pH 7.0	22	(19.0)	16	(38)
pH 4.0	9	(15.0)	21	(30)
pH 9.2	21	(14.0)	7	(28)
(Total)	(86)	(80.5)	(75)	(161)

$$\chi^2 \text{ value for overall fit to 1:1 ratio} = \frac{5.5^2}{80.5} \times 2 = 0.752$$

$$\text{Total } \chi^2 \text{ value} = 2 \left[\frac{1.5^2}{32.5} + \frac{3.0^2}{19.0} + \frac{6.0^2}{15.0} + \frac{7.0^2}{14.0} \right] = 12.885$$

Compute χ^2 for heterogeneity and display the results.

Sources of variation	Degrees of freedom	χ^2	P
Deviation for 1:1 ratio	1	0.752	> 0.1
Heterogeneity	3	12.133	< 0.01
(Total)	(4)	(12.885)	—

Having established highly-significant heterogeneity, re-examine the table and note that the frequencies for both pH 4.0 and pH 9.2 deviate markedly from expectation (χ^2 values 4.80 and 7.00 respectively). Also note that the frequencies for control and for pH 7.0 deviate little (χ^2 values 0.138 and 0.947 respectively). Further note that the deviations for pH 4.0 and pH 9.2 are in opposite directions. We conclude that vaginal pH does affect sex ratio in mice, acidity increasing the proportion of females and alkalinity the proportion of males.

7–5

	G	g	(Total)
H	123(a)	27(b)	(150)
h	30(c)	21(d)	(51)
(Total)	(153)	(48)	(201)

For G–g, $\chi^2 = \dfrac{1}{603}(153 - 144)^2 = 0.134$, with one degree of freedom, corresponding to $P > 0.5$.

For H–h, $\chi^2 = \dfrac{1}{603}(150 - 153)^2 = 0.015$, with one degree of freedom, corresponding to $P > 0.9$.

For linkage, $\chi^2 = \dfrac{1}{1809}(123 + 189 - 3 \times 57)^2 = \underline{10.99}$, with one degree of freedom, corresponding to $P < 0.001$.

We conclude that there is no significant deviation from the hypothesis of 3:1 segregation for G:g and H:h but that there is highly-significant linkage.

7–6 χ^2 for overall
segregation $= 2\left(340 \ln\dfrac{340}{360} + 140 \ln\dfrac{140}{120} \right)$

$= 4.29447$, with one degree of freedom

$$\chi^2 \text{ for batch 1} = 2\left(60 \ln\frac{60}{64.5} + 26 \ln\frac{26}{21.5}\right)$$

$$= 1.20379$$

χ^2 for batch 2 $= 1.70011$
χ^2 for batch 3 $= 2.63151$
χ^2 for batch 4 $= 8.53405$
χ^2 for batch 5 $= 0.35103$

Total χ^2 14.42049, with five degrees of freedom
less overall χ^2 4.29447, with one degree of freedom
heterogeneity χ^2 10.12602, with four degrees of freedom

(Check: heterogeneity χ^2 by method of $c \times r$ table $= 10.12602$.)

Chapter 8

8-1 $\Sigma X = $ 1107.3 $\Sigma Y = $ 60.22 $N = $ 20
$\Sigma X^2 = 61836.63$ $\Sigma Y^2 = 187.465$ $\Sigma XY = 3375.310$
$\Sigma x^2 = $ 530.9655 $\Sigma y^2 = $ 6.14258 $\Sigma xy = $ 41.2297

$$r = \frac{41.2297}{\sqrt{(530.9655 \times 6.14258)}} = 0.722, \text{with 18 degrees of}$$

freedom giving
$P < 0.001$

8-2 $\Sigma X = $ 48 $\Sigma Y = $ 117.6 $N = $ 6
$\Sigma X^2 = 454$ $\Sigma Y^2 = 2658.52$ $\Sigma XY = 1097.4$
$\Sigma x^2 = $ 70 $\Sigma y^2 = $ 353.56 $\Sigma xy = $ 156.6
$\overline{X} = $ 8.0 $\overline{Y} = $ 19.6

$$b = \frac{156.6}{70} = 2.237$$

$$a = 19.6 - (2.237 \times 8.0) = 1.70$$

$$Y = 1.70 + 2.237X$$

Regression SS $= 156.6^2/70 = 350.34$
Residual SS $= 353.56 - 350.34 = 3.22$
s_R^2 $= 3.22/4 = 0.805$ $\therefore s_R = 0.897$
S.E. of b $= 0.897/\sqrt{70} = 0.107$
95% limits of b are $2.237 \pm 2.776 \times 0.107$
± 0.298, i.e. 1.939 to 2.535

8-3 $\Sigma x^2 = 5.0238$ $\Sigma y^2 = 483.74$ $\Sigma xy = 42.835$
$\overline{X} = 1.023$ $\overline{Y} = $ 6.234

$$b = \frac{42.835}{5.0238} = 8.526$$

$$a = 6.234 - (8.526 \times 1.023) = -2.488$$

$$Y = 8.526X - 2.488$$

$$s_R{}^2 = \left(483.74 - \frac{42.835^2}{5.0238} \right)\Big/ 38 = 3.119 \quad \therefore \; s_R = 1.766$$

S.E. of $b = 1.766/\sqrt{5.0238} \qquad = 0.788$

$t = 8.526/0.788 = 10.82$, with 38 degrees of freedom,
giving $P < 0.001$

Tree height for 1% nitrogen $= 8.526 - 2.488 = 6.038$ m
95% confidence limits,

$$6.038 \pm 2.024 \times 1.766 \qquad \sqrt{\left(1 + \frac{1}{40} + \frac{0.023^2}{5.0238} \right)}$$

i.e. 6.038 ± 3.619 m

Chapter 9

9-1   Preliminary inspection of the results shows that there are some
large differences between treatment means suggesting the need
for a preliminary test of inequality of treatment variances.

	B	G	Y	R	F–R	F–W	I–W
s^2	0.4187	0.0937	0.3360	0.0377	0.1999	0.4217	0.4510

$$F_{max} = \frac{0.4510}{0.0377} = 11.96,\ \text{which is}\ < 20.8,\ \text{the tabulated value for}$$

seven treatments and five degrees of freedom per treatment. We
conclude that the sample variances do *not* differ significantly.

	B	G	Y	R	F–R	F–W	I–W
ΣX	33.80	36.10	100.20	113.50	24.63	127.60	128.10
$\overline{X}$	5.6333	6.0167	16.7000	18.9167	4.1050	21.2667˙	21.3500

$$GT = 563.93 \qquad \Sigma X^2 = 9787.4509$$
$$C = \frac{563.93^2}{42} = 7571.8344$$
$$SS = 9\,787.4509 - C = 2215.6165$$
$$SST = 9\,777.6578 - C = 2205.8234$$
$$SSE = 9.7931$$

Sources of variation	Sums-of-squares	Degrees of freedom	Mean-squares	F
Treatments	2205.8234	6	367.6372	1313.93***
Error	9.7931	35	0.2798	
(Total)	(2215.6165)	(41)		

The computed F value greatly exceeds the tabulated values for 6/30 and 6/40 degrees of freedom and $P = 0.001$ so we conclude that the differences between the treatments are very highly significant.

S.E. of treatment mean $= \sqrt{(0.2798/6)} = 0.21595$

Means	7	6	5	4	3	2	
Q's	4.43	4.27	4.08	3.82	3.46	2.88	
SSR's	0.957	0.922	0.881	0.825	0.747	0.622	
$\overline{X}$'s	4.105	5.633	6.017	16.700	18.917	21.267	21.350

9–2 $T_1 = 6.91$, $T_2 = 5.97$, $T_3 = 5.05$, $T_4 = 3.67$, GT $= 21.60$,
$\Sigma X^2 = 41.05$
$\quad C = 21.60^2/12 = 38.88$
$\quad SS = 41.05 - 38.88 = 2.17$
$SST = (6.91^2 + 5.97^2 + 5.05^2 + 3.67^2)/3 - C = 1.91$
$SSE = 2.17 - 1.91 = 0.26$

Sources of variation	Sums-of-squares	Degrees of freedom	Mean-squares	F
Fish	1.91	3	0.637	19.6***
Replicates	0.26	8	0.0325	—
(Total)	(2.17)	(11)	—	—

The computed F value exceeds the tabulated value for 3/8 degrees of freedom and $P = 0.001$ (15.8). We conclude that the variation between fish is greater than can be accounted for by variation between replicates, or more exactly, that there is a very highly significant extra variance component between fish. (For a method of computing actual variance components see SNEDECOR and COCHRAN (1967) section 10.13 or SOKAL and ROHLF (1979), Box 9.3.)

9–3

	C	E	M
$\overline{X}$	5.873	5.791	5.628

$C = 739.00^2/128 = 4266.5703$
$SS = 4273.5345 - C = 6.9642$
$SST = 281.91^2/48 + 243.24^2/42 + 213.85^2/38 - C = 1.2985$
$SSE = 6.9642 - 1.2985 = 5.6657$

Sources of variation	Sums-of-squares	Degrees of freedom	Mean-squares	F
Cover types	1.2985	2	0.6493	14.33***
Error	5.6657	125	0.0453	—
(Total)	(6.9642)	(127)	—	—

The computed value of F greatly exceeds the tabulated value of F for 2/120 degrees of freedom and $P = 0.001$ (7.32) so we conclude that the effect of cover type on soil surface pH is very highly significant.

As both C and E are ericaceous shrubs it would seem appropriate to make two independent comparisons: between the shrubs (taken together) and the moss, and between the two shrubs.

$SS_{shrubs/moss} = (281.91 + 243.24)^2/90 + 213.85^2/38 - C$
$= 1.1490$
$SS_{btn\ shrubs} = 1.2985 - 1.1490 = 0.1495$

Sources of variation	Sums-of-squares	Degrees of freedom	Mean-squares	F
Cover types	1.2985	2	(0.6493)	
shrubs/moss	1.1490	1	1.1490	25.36***
btn shrubs	0.1495	1	0.1495	3.30 NS
Error	5.6657	125	0.0453	

The computed F value for shrubs/moss greatly exceeds the tabulated value of F for 1/120 degrees of freedom and $P = 0.001$ (11.4) so we conclude that the pH difference between moss and the two shrubs is very highly significant but the computed value for between shrubs is *less than* the tabulated value for $P = 0.05$ (3.07) so we conclude that the pH difference between shrubs is not significant.

9-4

$$C = \frac{190.874^2}{50} = 728.6577$$

$$SS = 730.194 - C = 1.5363$$

$$SST = 729.2428 - C = 0.5851$$

$$SSE = 1.5363 - 0.5851 = 0.9512$$

Sources of variation	Sums-of-squares	Degrees of freedom	Mean-squares	F
Treatments	0.5851	4	0.1463	6.92***
Error	0.9512	45	0.02114	—
(Total)	(1.5363)	(49)	—	—

This value of F exceeds the tabulated value of F for 4/45 degrees of freedom and $P = 0.001$ (5.57) so the differences between the treatments are very highly significant.

(a) L.S.D. $= 2.014 \sqrt{(2 \times 0.02114/10)} = 0.131$ (2.014 = t, for $P = 0.05$ and 45 degrees of freedom). The mean transformed value for red light (3.604) differs by more than the L.S.D. from the mean of each other treatment.

(b) L.S.R. $= 4.02 \sqrt{(0.02114/10)} = 0.185 (4.02 = Q$, for $P = 0.05$ and 45 degrees of freedom). The conclusion is the same as for the L.S.D. The tests will not always lead to the same conclusion: note that the L.S.R. is substantially larger than the L.S.D.

It could be argued that it would be more appropriate to compare the mean for red light with the mean for all the other treatments *taken together*, thus:

$$SS_{red/others} = 36.037^2/10 + 154.837^2/40 - C = 0.5713$$

$$SS_{others} = 0.5851 - 0.5713 = 0.0138$$

Sources of variation	Sums-of-squares	Degrees of freedom	Mean-squares	F
Treatments	0.5851	4	0.1463	(6.92)
red/others	0.5713	1	0.5713	27.02***
others	0.0138	3	0.0046	0.22 NS
Error	0.951 22	45	0.021 14	—
(Total)	(1.5363)	(49)	—	—

We conclude that the difference between the mean for red light and that for all other treatments taken together is very highly

significant but that the differences between the means for the
other treatments are non-significant.

9–5 $\Sigma y^2 = 353.56$; Regression SS $= 350.34$; Residual SS $= 3.22$.

Sources of variation	Sums-of-squares	Degrees of freedom	Mean-squares	F
Regression	350.34	1	350.34	435.2***
Residual	3.22	4	0.805	—
(Total)	(353.56)	(5)	—	—

The computed F value exceeds the tabulated value for 1/4 degrees
of freedom and $P = 0.001$ (74.1) so we conclude that the linear
component in the relationship is very highly significant.

9–6

Days	3	5	7	9	10	13	15	Total
ΣY	46	78	105	138	160	178	185	(890)
ΣY^2	354	1014	1839	3180	4270	5282	5705	(21 644)
$\bar{Y}$	7.67	13.00	17.50	23.00	26.67	29.67	30.83	

$$C = 890^2/42 = 18\,859.52$$
$$SS = 21\,644 - C = 2784.48$$
$$SST = 21\,629.67 - C = 2770.15$$
$$SSE = 2784.48 - 2770.15 = 14.33$$

$$\Sigma X = 378 \qquad \Sigma Y = 890 \qquad\qquad n = 42$$
$$\Sigma X^2 = 4074 \qquad \Sigma Y^2 = 21\,644 \qquad \Sigma XY = 9354$$
$$\Sigma x^2 = 672 \qquad \Sigma y^2 = 2784.48 \qquad \Sigma xy = 1344$$
$$\bar{X} = 9.00 \qquad\quad \bar{Y} = 21.19$$
$$b = 1344/672 = 2.00$$
$$a = 21.19 - (2.00 \times 9.00) = 3.19$$
$$Y = 3.19 + 2.00\,X$$

Regression SS $= 1344^2/672 = 2688.00$

Sources of variation	Sums-of-squares	Degrees of freedom	Mean-squares	F
Treatments	2770.15	6	461.69	
Regression	2688.00	1	2688.00	163.60***
Deviation	82.15	5	16.43	40.13***
Error	14.33	35	0.4094	—
(Total)	(2784.48)	(41)	—	—

Deviation MS over Error MS gives $F = 40.13$ with 5/35 degrees of freedom and $P < 0.001$. *Regression MS over Deviation MS* gives $F = 163.60$ with 1/5 degrees of freedom and $P < 0.001$. We conclude that the relationship between colony diameter and time has a very highly significant rectilinear component but shows very highly significant deviation from linearity. Examination of a plot of mean diameter against time indicates that by day 13 the growth rate has begun to fall.

(NB   In such an analysis if F for Deviation is less than unity a pooled estimate of error may be computed, provided that the conditions in section 10.3 (ix) (c) are satisfied.)

9-7

10 mg l^{-1}	20 mg l^{-1}

$\Sigma X = 24$

$\Sigma X^2 = 164$

$\Sigma x^2 = 20$

$\overline{X} = 6$

10 mg l^{-1}:
$\Sigma Y = 42.7 \qquad n = 4$
$\Sigma Y^2 = 513.49 \quad \Sigma XY = 290.1$
$\Sigma y^2 = 57.67 \quad \Sigma xy = 33.9$
$\overline{Y} = 10.675$
$b = 33.9/20 = 1.695$
$a = 10.675 - (1.695 \times 6)$
$\quad = 0.505$
$Y = 0.505 + 1.695 \, X$

20 mg l^{-1}:
$\Sigma Y = 53.5 \qquad n = 4$
$\Sigma Y^2 = 815.73 \quad \Sigma XY = 365.7$
$\Sigma y^2 = 100.17 \quad \Sigma xy = 44.7$
$\overline{Y} = 13.38$
$b = 44.7/20 = 2.235$
$a = 13.38 - (2.235 \times 6)$
$\quad = -0.03$
$Y = -0.035 + 2.235 \, X$

Regression SS $= 33.9^2/20 = 57.46$; $\quad = 44.7^2/20 = 99.90$

Residual SS $= 57.67 - 57.46 = 0.21$; $\quad = 100.17 - 99.90 = 0.27$

Residual MS $= 0.21/2 = 0.105$; $\quad = 0.27/2 = 0.135$

$F = 0.135/0.105 = 1.286$, with 2/2 degrees of freedom, giving (for a 2-tailed test) $P > 0.5$

	df	Σx^2	Σxy	Σy^2	b	Deviation from regression df	S—S	M—S
10 mg l^{-1}	3	20	33.9	57.67	1.695	2	0.21	—
20 mg l^{-1}	3	20	44.7	100.17	2.235	2	0.27	—
					Total	4 (i)	0.48	0.12
Pooled	6	40	78.6	157.84	1.965	5 (ii)	3.39	—
					Difference	1 (iii)	2.91	2.91

(NB Residual SS, pooled data $= 157.84 - (78.6^2/40)$.)

$F = 2.91/0.12 = 24.25$, with 1/4 degrees of freedom, giving $P < 0.01$. We conclude that there is a highly significant difference between regression coefficients, i.e. linear growth rates.

Chapter 10

10-1

Block	1	2	3	4	5	6
Block totals	93.30	94.05	96.05	95.30	92.43	92.80

$\text{SSB} = 7573.3043 - C = 1.4699$

$\text{SSE} = 2215.6165 - (2205.8234 + 1.4699) = 8.3232$

Sources of variation	Sums-of-squares	Degrees of freedom	Mean-squares	F
Treatments	2205.8234	6	367.6372	1325.3***
Students (blocks)	1.4699	5	0.2940	1.06 NS
Error	8.3232	30	0.2774	—
(Total)	(2215.6165)	(41)	—	—

The F value for between students is very close to unity so there is no evidence of systematic error associated with students. The MSE is changed so little that the previous comparisons between treatment means remain unaffected.

10–2 First compute sub-class, treatment, block and grand totals.

Fish	NaCN −	NaCN +	(Total)
1	5.72	3.56	(9.28)
2	5.45	3.97	(9.42)
3	3.25	2.49	(5.74)
4	4.88	3.37	(8.25)
(Total)	(19.30)	(13.39)	(32.69)

$$C = 32.69^2/24 = 44.5265$$
$$SS = (1.54^2 + 1.92^2 + 2.26^2 + 1.10^2 + ... + 1.32^2) - C = 3.8166$$
$$SSQ = (5.72^2 + 5.45^2 + 3.25^2 + ... 3.37^2)/3 - C = 3.0699$$
$$SSE = 3.8166 - 3.0699 = 0.7467$$
$$SST = (19.30^2 + 13.39^2)/12 - C = 1.4553$$
$$SSB = (9.28^2 + 9.42^2 + 5.74^2 + 8.25^2)/6 - C = 1.4510$$
$$SSTB = 3.0699 - (1.4553 + 1.4510) = 0.1636$$

Sources of variation	Sums-of-squares	Degrees of freedom	Mean-squares	F
Treatments	1.4553	1	1.4553	26.70*
Fish	1.4510	3	0.4837	10.36***
Interaction	0.1636	3	0.0545	1.17 NS
Error	0.7467	16	0.0467	—
(Total)	(3.8166)	(23)	—	—

F for interaction, with 3/16 degrees of freedom gives $P > 0.25$ so we conclude that interaction is not significant. Testing MSB/MSE: F for fish is 10.36 with 3/16 degrees of freedom, giving $P < 0.001$, thereby justifying the use of the randomized-block design. Testing MST/MSI: F for treatments is 26.70 with 1/3 degrees of freedom, giving $P < 0.05$.
The difference between the treatment means, $(19.30-13.29)/12 = 0.49$ is thus significant.

95% confidence limits of the difference

$$= 3.182 \sqrt{\left(\frac{2 \times 0.0545}{12} \right)} = 0.30$$

Thus: the addition of NaCN to the medium reduced the uptake of amino acid by $0.49 \pm 0.30\ \mu\mathrm{mol\ g^{-1}}$ dry weight 20 $\mathrm{min^{-1}}$ period.

10-3

$C = 7213^2/80 = 650\,342$
$SS = 830\,327 - C = 179\,985$
$SST = (2986^2 + 4227^2)/40 - C = 669\,593 - C = 19\,251$
$SSB = (5249^2 + 1964^2)/40 - C = 785\,232 - C = 134\,890$
$SSQ = (2255^2 + 2994^2 + 731^2 + 1233^2)/20 - C = 805\,186 - C$
$\qquad = 154\,844$
$SSE = 179\,985 - 154\,844 = 25\,141$
$SSTB = 154\,844 - (19\,251 + 134\,890) = 703$

Sources of variation	Sums-of-squares	Degrees of freedom	Mean-squares	F
Ethanol	19 251	1	19 251	58.16***
Acetaldehyde	134 890	1	134 890	407.5***
Interaction	703	1	703	2.124 NS
Error	25 141	76	331	—
(Total)	(179 985)	(99)	—	—

F for interaction, with 1/76 degrees of freedom, is 2.124, giving $P > 0.1$. We conclude that interaction is non-significant and test for main effects. F values, again with 1/76 degrees of freedom, of 58.16 for ethanol and 407.5 for acetaldehyde both give $P < 0.001$. We conclude that the effects of both ethanol and acetaldehyde are very highly significant.

Effect of ethanol
Difference in means $= 31.0$; $s^2 = 331$, so $s = 18.19$

S.E. of difference $= s \sqrt{(1/40 + 1/40)} = 4.07$
95% limits of difference are $31.0 \pm 2.0 \times 4.07$
i.e. 31.0 ± 8.14
Therefore 80 ppm ethanol *increases* gametophyte length by 31.0 ± 8.14 units.

Effect of acetaldehyde
Difference in means $= 82.1$
95% limits of difference are 82.1 ± 8.14
Therefore 20 ppm acetaldehyde *decreases* gametophyte length by 82.1 ± 8.14 units.

10–4

$C = 224.321^2/80 = 629.00$
$SS = 687 - C = 58$
$SST = (114.315^2 + 110.006^2)/40 - C = 629.23 - C = 0.23$
$SSB = (138.295^2 + 86.026^2)/40 - C = 663.15 - C = 34.15$
$SSQ = (76.281^2 + 62.014^2 + 38.034^2 + 37.992^2)/20 - C = 41.72$
$SSE = 58 - 41.72 = 16.28$
$SSTB = 41.72 - (0.23 + 34.15) = 7.34$

Sources of variation	Sums-of-squares	Degrees of freedom	Mean-squares	F
Ethanol	0.23	1	0.23	—
Acetaldehyde	34.15	1	34.15	—
Interaction	7.34	1	7.34	34.27***
Error	16.28	76	0.2142	—
(Total)	(58.00)	(79)	—	—

F for interaction, with 1/76 degrees of freedom, is 34.27 giving $P < 0.001$. We therefore conclude that interaction is very-highly significant. Set up a table of sub-class totals, thus:

		−	*Ethanol*	+
	O	3.814	3.101	(6.915)
−	E	3.515	3.407	
	Diff	+0.303	−0.303	
Acetaldehyde				
	O	1.902	2.400	(4.302)
+	E	2.205	2.097	
	Diff	−0.303	+0.303	
		(5.716)	(5.501)	(11.217)

Both substances appear to reduce cell number, strictly $\sqrt{}$(cell number). In combination they have less effect than would be expected, i.e. they show *negative interaction*, and this is very-highly significant. To make statements about the effects of ethanol and acetaldehyde, extract the data for two separate experiments; $\pm$ ethanol and $\pm$ acetaldehyde.

Ethanol

$C = 138.295^2/40 = 478.138$

$SS = 492 - C = 13.862$

$SST = (76.281^2 + 62.014^2)/20 - C = 483.226 - C = 5.088$

$SSE = 13.862 - 5.088 = 8.774$

Sources of variation	Sums-of-squares	Degrees of freedom	Mean-squares	F
Ethanol	5.088	1	5.088	22.04***
Error	8.774	38	0.2309	—
(Total)	(13.862)	(39)	—	—

F, with 1/38 degrees of freedom, is 22.04, giving $P < 0.001$. Attach 95% confidence limits to treatment means.

Ethanol $-$: $\overline{X} = 3.814$; $s^2 = 0.2309$.

S.E. of $\overline{X} = \sqrt{(0.2309/20)} = 0.10745$

95% limits of $\overline{X}$ are $3.814 \pm 2.02 \times 0.10745$

i.e. 3.814 ± 0.217

i.e. 4.031 to 3.597

Back-transforming (X^2) 16.25 to 12.94 cells

Ethanol $+$: $\overline{X} = 3.101$

95% limits of $\overline{X}$ are 3.101 ± 0.217

i.e. 3.318 to 2.884

Back-transforming (X^2) 11.01 to 8.32 cells

Acetaldehyde

$C = 114.315^2/40 = 326.698$

$SS = 371 - C = 44.302$

$SST = (76.281^2 + 38.034^2)20 - C = 363.269 - C = 36.571$

$SSE = 44.302 - 36.571 = 7.731$

Sources of variation	Sums-of-squares	Degrees of freedom	Mean-squares	F
Acetaldehyde	36.571	1	36.571	179.79***
Error	7.731	38	0.2034	—
(Total)	(44.302)	(39)	—	—

F, with $1/38$ degrees of freedom is 179.79, giving $P < 0.001$. Attach 95% confidence limits to treatment means.

Acetaldehyde $-$: $\overline{X} = 3.841$; $s^2 = 0.2034$

S.E. of $\overline{X} = \sqrt{(0.2034/20)} = 0.10085$

95% limits of $\overline{X}$ are $3.841 \pm 2.02 \times 0.10085$
　　　　　i.e. 3.841 ± 0.204
　　　　　i.e. 4.045 to 3.637
Back-transforming (X^2) 16.36 to 13.23 cells

Acetaldehyde $+$: $\overline{X} = 1.902$
95% limits of $\overline{X}$ are 1.902 ± 0.204
　　　　　i.e. 2.105 to 1.698
Back-transforming (X^2) 4.44 to 2.88 cells

(NB As no doubt has been shown on the equality of the variance between replicates within the four sub-classes confidence limits to treatment means could have been estimated using the mean-square for error of the whole data, i.e. 0.2142 and t with 76 degrees of freedom.)

10–5　$C = 2122.4^2/108 = 41709.090$
$SST = (730.9^2 + 674.0^2 + 717.5^2)/36 - C = 49.162$
SS litters $= 42434.713 - C = 725.623$
SS offspring $= 42495.950 - C = 786.870$
SS litters within treatments $= 725.623 - 49.162 = 676.461$
SS offpring in litters $= 786.870 - 725.623 = 61.247$

Sources of variation	Sums-of-squares	Degrees of freedom	Mean-squares	F
Treatments	49.162	2	24.581	1.20 NS
Litters within treatments	676.461	33	20.499	24.10***
Offspring in litters	61.247	72	0.85065	—

We conclude that the differences between treatment means are not significant and that there is a very highly significant additional variance component between litters.

Ignoring the classification into litters is the same as computing a pooled MS for between offspring, thus:

MSE = (676.461 + 61.247)/(33 + 72) = 7.0258
This would give F for treatments 24.581/7.0258 = 3.50*, and the conclusion drawn would be incorrect.

10–6 Row totals: (1) 147; (2) 151; (3) 144; (4) 152; (5) 150; (6) 146

SSB = $(147^2 + 151^2 + \ldots 146^2)/7 - C = 7.05$

SSE = $2784.48 - (2770.15 + 7.05) = 7.28$

Sources of variation	Sums-of-squares	Degrees of freedom	Mean-squares	F
Treatments	2770.15	6	461.69	—
Regression	2688.00	1	2688.00	163.60***
Remainder	82.15	5	16.43	67.70***
Blocks	7.05	5	1.41	5.81***
Error	7.28	30	0.2427	—
(Total)	(2784.48)	(41)	—	—

F for blocks (5.81) with 5/30 degrees of freedom gives $P < 0.001$, so we conclude that there are very highly significant differences between colonies. This means that some colonies were consistently larger than the mean and others consistently smaller, throughout the time period. The MSE has been decreased and the F value for deviations increased but in this case the conclusions remain the same.

Further Reading

BAILEY, N. T. (1959). *Statistical Methods in Biology*. English Universities Press, London.

CAMPBELL, R. C. (1974). *Statistics for Biologists*. 2nd. edn., Cambridge University Press, London.

CLARKE G. M. (1969). *Statistics and Experimental Design*. Edward Arnold, London.

HEATH, O. V. S. (1970). *Investigation by Experiment*. Studies in Biology no. 23, Edward Arnold, London.

MATHER, K. (1949). *Statistical Analysis in Biology*. Methuen, London.

MATHER, K. (1967). *The Elements of Biometry*. Methuen, London.

SNEDECOR G. W. and COCHRAN W. G. (1967). *Statistical Methods*. 6th edn., Iowa State University Press.

SOKAL, R. R. and ROHLF, F. J. (1969). *Biometry*. Freeman, London.

SOKAL, R. R. and ROHLF, F. J. (1973). *Introduction to Biostatistics*. Freeman, London.

Statistical tables

FISHER, R. A. and YATES, F. (1963). *Statistical Tables for Biological, Agricultural and Medical Research*, Oliver and Boyd, Edinburgh.

LINDLEY, D. V. and MILLER, J. C. P. (1968). *Cambridge Elementary Statistical Tables*. Cambridge University Press, London.

PEARSON, E. S. and HARTLEY, H. O. (1962). *Biometrika Tables for Statisticians*. Vol. 1, Cambridge University Press, London.

ROHLF, F. J. and SOKAL, R. R. (1969). *Statistical Tables*. Freeman, London.

Selected Statistical Tables

Table 1 Student's *t*. Values exceeded with probability *p*

d.f.	$p = 0.1$	0.05	0.02	0.01	0.002	0.001
1	6.314	12.706	31.821	63.657	318.31	636.62
2	2.920	4.303	6.965	9.925	22.327	31.598
3	2.353	3.182	4.541	5.841	10.214	12.924
4	2.132	2.776	3.747	4.604	7.173	8.610
5	2.015	2.571	3.365	4.032	5.893	6.869
6	1.943	2.447	3.143	3.707	5.208	5.959
7	1.895	2.365	2.998	3.499	4.785	5.408
8	1.860	2.306	2.896	3.355	4.501	5.041
9	1.833	2.262	2.821	3.250	4.297	4.781
10	1.812	2.228	2.764	3.169	4.144	4.587
11	1.796	2.201	2.718	3.106	4.025	4.437
12	1.782	2.179	2.681	3.055	3.930	4.318
13	1.771	2.160	2.650	3.012	3.852	4.221
14	1.761	2.145	2.624	2.977	3.787	4.140
15	1.753	2.131	2.602	2.947	3.733	4.073
16	1.746	2.120	2.583	2.921	3.686	4.015
17	1.740	2.110	2.567	2.898	3.646	3.965
18	1.734	2.101	2.552	2.878	3.610	3.922
19	1.729	2.093	2.539	2.861	3.579	3.883
20	1.725	2.086	2.528	2.845	3.552	3.850
21	1.721	2.080	2.518	2.831	3.527	3.819
22	1.717	2.074	2.508	2.819	3.505	3.792
23	1.714	2.069	2.500	2.807	3.485	3.767
24	1.711	2.064	2.492	2.797	3.467	3.745
25	1.708	2.060	2.485	2.787	3.450	3.725
26	1.706	2.056	2.479	2.779	3.435	3.707
27	1.703	2.052	2.473	2.771	3.421	3.690
28	1.701	2.048	2.467	2.763	3.408	3.674
29	1.699	2.045	2.462	2.756	3.396	3.659
30	1.697	2.042	2.457	2.750	3.385	3.646
40	1.684	2.021	2.423	2.704	3.307	3.551
60	1.671	2.000	2.390	2.660	3.232	3.460
120	1.658	1.980	2.358	2.617	3.160	3.373
∞	1.645	1.960	2.326	2.576	3.090	3.291

The last row of the table (∞) gives values of d, the 'standardized normal deviate'. (Tables 1 to 4 are reproduced by permission of the Trustees, from *Biometrika Tables for Statisticians*, 3rd Edition (1966), ed. E. S. Pearson and H. O. Hartley)

Table 2 χ^2

d.f.	$p = 0.900$	0.500	0.100	0.050	0.010	0.001
1	0.016	0.455	2.71	3.84	6.63	10.83
2	0.211	1.39	4.61	5.99	9.21	13.82
3	0.584	2.37	6.25	7.81	11.34	16.27
4	1.06	3.36	7.78	9.49	13.28	18.47
5	1.61	4.35	9.24	11.07	15.09	20.52
6	2.20	5.35	10.64	12.59	16.81	22.46
7	2.83	6.35	12.02	14.07	18.48	24.32
8	3.49	7.34	13.36	15.51	20.09	26.13
9	4.17	8.34	14.68	16.92	21.67	27.88
10	4.87	9.34	15.99	18.31	23.21	29.59
11	5.58	10.34	17.28	19.68	24.73	31.26
12	6.30	11.34	18.55	21.03	26.22	32.91
13	7.04	12.34	19.81	22.36	27.69	34.53
14	7.79	13.34	21.06	23.68	29.14	36.12
15	8.55	14.34	22.31	25.00	30.58	37.70
16	9.31	15.34	23.54	26.30	32.00	39.25
17	10.09	16.34	24.77	27.59	33.41	40.79
18	10.86	17.34	25.99	28.87	34.81	42.31
19	11.65	18.34	27.20	30.14	36.19	43.82
20	12.44	19.34	28.41	31.41	37.57	45.32
21	13.24	20.34	29.62	32.67	38.93	46.80
22	14.04	21.34	30.81	33.92	40.29	48.27
23	14.85	22.34	32.01	35.17	41.64	49.73
24	15.66	23.34	33.20	36.42	42.98	51.18
25	16.47	24.34	34.38	37.65	44.31	52.62
26	17.29	25.34	33.56	38.89	45.64	54.05
27	18.11	26.34	36.74	40.11	46.96	55.48
28	18.94	27.34	37.92	41.34	48.28	56.89
29	19.77	28.34	39.09	42.56	49.59	58.30
30	20.60	29.34	40.26	43.77	50.89	59.70
40	29.05	39.34	51.81	55.76	63.69	73.40
50	37.69	49.33	63.17	67.50	76.15	86.66
60	46.46	59.33	74.40	79.08	88.38	99.61
70	55.33	69.33	85.53	90.53	100.43	112.32
80	64.28	79.33	96.58	101.88	112.33	124.84
90	73.29	89.33	107.57	113.15	124.12	137.21
100	82.36	99.33	118.50	123.34	135.81	149.45

Table 3   The correlation coefficient, r

d.f.	$p = 0.1$	0.05	0.02	0.01	0.005	0.001
1	0.9877	0.9^2692	0.9^3507	0.9^3877	0.9^4692	0.9^5877
2	0.9000	0.9500	0.9800	0.9^2000	0.9^2500	0.9^3000
3	0.805	0.878	0.9343	0.9587	0.9740	0.9^2114
4	0.729	0.811	0.882	0.9172	0.9417	0.9741
5	0.669	0.754	0.833	0.875	0.9056	0.9509
6	0.621	0.707	0.789	0.834	0.870	0.9249
7	0.582	0.666	0.750	0.798	0.836	0.898
8	0.549	0.632	0.715	0.765	0.805	0.872
9	0.521	0.602	0.685	0.735	0.776	0.847
10	0.497	0.576	0.658	0.708	0.750	0.823
11	0.476	0.553	0.634	0.684	0.726	0.801
12	0.457	0.532	0.612	0.661	0.703	0.780
13	0.441	0.514	0.592	0.641	0.683	0.760
14	0.426	0.497	0.574	0.623	0.664	0.742
15	0.412	0.482	0.558	0.606	0.647	0.725
16	0.400	0.468	0.543	0.590	0.631	0.708
17	0.389	0.456	0.529	0.575	0.616	0.693
18	0.378	0.444	0.516	0.561	0.602	0.679
19	0.369	0.433	0.503	0.549	0.589	0.665
20	0.360	0.423	0.492	0.537	0.576	0.652
25	0.323	0.381	0.445	0.487	0.524	0.597
30	0.296	0.349	0.409	0.449	0.484	0.554
35	0.275	0.325	0.381	0.418	0.452	0.519
40	0.257	0.304	0.358	0.393	0.425	0.490
45	0.243	0.288	0.338	0.372	0.403	0.465
50	0.231	0.273	0.322	0.354	0.384	0.443
60	0.211	0.250	0.295	0.325	0.352	0.408
70	0.195	0.232	0.274	0.302	0.327	0.380
80	0.183	0.217	0.257	0.283	0.307	0.357
90	0.173	0.205	0.242	0.267	0.290	0.338
100	0.164	0.195	0.230	0.254	0.276	0.321

$$\text{d.f.} = (N - 2)$$

Table 4 The variance ratio, F $p = 0.05$

v_2 \ v_1	1	2	3	4	5	6	7	8	9	10	12	15	20	24	30	40	60	120	∞
1	161.4	199.5	215.7	224.6	230.2	234.0	236.8	238.9	240.5	241.9	243.9	245.9	248.0	249.1	250.1	251.1	252.2	253.3	254.3
2	18.51	19.00	19.16	19.25	19.30	19.33	19.35	19.37	19.38	19.40	19.41	19.43	19.45	19.45	19.46	19.47	19.48	19.49	19.50
3	10.13	9.55	9.28	9.12	9.01	8.94	8.89	8.85	8.81	8.79	8.74	8.70	8.66	8.64	8.62	8.59	8.57	8.55	8.53
4	7.71	6.94	6.59	6.39	6.26	6.16	6.09	6.04	6.00	5.96	5.91	5.86	5.80	5.77	5.75	5.72	5.69	5.66	5.63
5	6.61	5.79	5.41	5.19	5.05	4.95	4.88	4.82	4.77	4.74	4.68	4.62	4.56	4.53	4.50	4.46	4.43	4.40	4.36
6	5.99	5.14	4.76	4.53	4.39	4.28	4.21	4.15	4.10	4.06	4.00	3.94	3.87	3.84	3.81	3.77	3.74	3.70	3.67
7	5.59	4.74	4.35	4.12	3.97	3.87	3.79	3.73	3.68	3.64	3.57	3.51	3.44	3.41	3.38	3.34	3.30	3.27	3.23
8	5.32	4.46	4.07	3.84	3.69	3.58	3.50	3.44	3.39	3.35	3.28	3.22	3.15	3.12	3.08	3.04	3.01	2.97	2.93
9	5.12	4.26	3.86	3.63	3.48	3.37	3.29	3.23	3.18	3.14	3.07	3.01	2.94	2.90	2.86	2.83	2.79	2.75	2.71
10	4.96	4.10	3.71	3.48	3.33	3.22	3.14	3.07	3.02	2.98	2.91	2.85	2.77	2.74	2.70	2.66	2.62	2.58	2.54
11	4.84	3.98	3.59	3.36	3.20	3.09	3.01	2.95	2.90	2.85	2.79	2.72	2.65	2.61	2.57	2.53	2.49	2.45	2.40
12	4.75	3.89	3.49	3.26	3.11	3.00	2.91	2.85	2.80	2.75	2.69	2.62	2.54	2.51	2.47	2.43	2.38	2.34	2.30
13	4.67	3.81	3.41	3.18	3.03	2.92	2.83	2.77	2.71	2.67	2.60	2.53	2.46	2.42	2.38	2.34	2.30	2.25	2.21
14	4.60	3.74	3.34	3.11	2.96	2.85	2.76	2.70	2.65	2.60	2.53	2.46	2.39	2.35	2.31	2.27	2.22	2.18	2.13
15	4.54	3.68	3.29	3.06	2.90	2.79	2.71	2.64	2.59	2.54	2.48	2.40	2.33	2.29	2.25	2.20	2.16	2.11	2.07
16	4.49	3.63	3.24	3.01	2.85	2.74	2.66	2.59	2.54	2.49	2.42	2.35	2.28	2.24	2.19	2.15	2.11	2.06	2.01
17	4.45	3.59	3.20	2.96	2.81	2.70	2.61	2.55	2.49	2.45	2.38	2.31	2.23	2.19	2.15	2.10	2.06	2.01	1.96
18	4.41	3.55	3.16	2.93	2.77	2.66	2.58	2.51	2.46	2.41	2.34	2.27	2.19	2.15	2.11	2.06	2.02	1.97	1.92
19	4.38	3.52	3.13	2.90	2.74	2.63	2.54	2.48	2.42	2.38	2.31	2.23	2.16	2.11	2.07	2.03	1.98	1.93	1.88
20	4.35	3.49	3.10	2.87	2.71	2.60	2.51	2.45	2.39	2.35	2.28	2.20	2.12	2.08	2.04	1.99	1.95	1.90	1.84
21	4.32	3.47	3.07	2.84	2.68	2.57	2.49	2.42	2.37	2.32	2.25	2.18	2.10	2.05	2.01	1.96	1.92	1.87	1.81
22	4.30	3.44	3.05	2.82	2.66	2.55	2.46	2.40	2.34	2.30	2.23	2.15	2.07	2.03	1.98	1.94	1.89	1.84	1.78
23	4.28	3.42	3.03	2.80	2.64	2.53	2.44	2.37	2.32	2.27	2.20	2.13	2.05	2.01	1.96	1.91	1.86	1.81	1.76
24	4.26	3.40	3.01	2.78	2.62	2.51	2.42	2.36	2.30	2.25	2.18	2.11	2.03	1.98	1.94	1.89	1.84	1.79	1.73
25	4.24	3.39	2.99	2.76	2.60	2.49	2.40	2.34	2.28	2.24	2.16	2.09	2.01	1.96	1.92	1.87	1.82	1.77	1.71
26	4.23	3.37	2.98	2.74	2.59	2.47	2.39	2.32	2.27	2.22	2.15	2.07	1.99	1.95	1.90	1.85	1.80	1.75	1.69
27	4.21	3.35	2.96	2.73	2.57	2.46	2.37	2.31	2.25	2.20	2.13	2.06	1.97	1.93	1.88	1.84	1.79	1.73	1.67
28	4.20	3.34	2.95	2.71	2.56	2.45	2.36	2.29	2.24	2.19	2.12	2.04	1.96	1.91	1.87	1.82	1.77	1.71	1.65
29	4.18	3.33	2.93	2.70	2.55	2.43	2.35	2.28	2.22	2.18	2.10	2.03	1.94	1.90	1.85	1.81	1.75	1.70	1.64
30	4.17	3.32	2.92	2.69	2.53	2.42	2.33	2.27	2.21	2.16	2.09	2.01	1.93	1.89	1.84	1.79	1.74	1.68	1.62
40	4.08	3.23	2.84	2.61	2.45	2.34	2.25	2.18	2.12	2.08	2.00	1.92	1.84	1.79	1.74	1.69	1.64	1.58	1.51
60	4.00	3.15	2.76	2.53	2.37	2.25	2.17	2.10	2.04	1.99	1.92	1.84	1.75	1.70	1.65	1.59	1.53	1.47	1.39
120	3.92	3.07	2.68	2.45	2.29	2.17	2.09	2.02	1.96	1.91	1.83	1.75	1.66	1.61	1.55	1.50	1.43	1.35	1.25
∞	3.84	3.00	2.60	2.37	2.21	2.10	2.01	1.94	1.88	1.83	1.75	1.67	1.57	1.52	1.46	1.39	1.32	1.22	1.00

$V_1 V_2$ are upper, lower d.f. respectively.

Table 4 (*cont.*) $p = 0.01$

v_2\\v_1	1	2	3	4	5	6	7	8	9	10	12	15	20	24	30	40	60	120	∞
1	4052	4999.5	5403	5625	5764	5859	5928	5982	6022	6056	6106	6157	6209	6235	6261	6287	6313	6339	6366
2	98.50	99.00	99.17	99.25	99.30	99.33	99.36	99.37	99.39	99.40	99.42	99.43	99.45	99.46	99.47	99.47	99.48	99.49	99.50
3	34.12	30.82	29.46	28.71	28.24	27.91	27.67	27.49	27.35	27.23	27.05	26.87	26.69	26.60	26.50	26.41	26.32	26.22	26.13
4	21.20	18.00	16.69	15.98	15.52	15.21	14.98	14.80	14.66	14.55	14.37	14.20	14.02	13.93	13.84	13.75	13.65	13.56	13.46
5	16.26	13.27	12.06	11.39	10.97	10.67	10.46	10.29	10.16	10.05	9.89	9.72	9.55	9.47	9.38	9.29	9.20	9.11	9.02
6	13.75	10.92	9.78	9.15	8.75	8.47	8.26	8.10	7.98	7.87	7.72	7.56	7.40	7.31	7.23	7.14	7.06	6.97	6.88
7	12.25	9.55	8.45	7.85	7.46	7.19	6.99	6.84	6.72	6.62	6.47	6.31	6.16	6.07	5.99	5.91	5.82	5.74	5.65
8	11.26	8.65	7.59	7.01	6.63	6.37	6.18	6.03	5.91	5.81	5.67	5.52	5.36	5.28	5.20	5.12	5.03	4.95	4.86
9	10.56	8.02	6.99	6.42	6.06	5.80	5.61	5.47	5.35	5.26	5.11	4.96	4.81	4.73	4.65	4.57	4.48	4.40	4.31
10	10.04	7.56	6.55	5.99	5.64	5.39	5.20	5.06	4.94	4.85	4.71	4.56	4.41	4.33	4.25	4.17	4.08	4.00	3.91
11	9.65	7.21	6.22	5.67	5.32	5.07	4.89	4.74	4.63	4.54	4.40	4.25	4.10	4.02	3.94	3.86	3.78	3.69	3.60
12	9.33	6.93	5.95	5.41	5.06	4.82	4.64	4.50	4.39	4.30	4.16	4.01	3.86	3.78	3.70	3.62	3.54	3.45	3.36
13	9.07	6.70	5.74	5.21	4.86	4.62	4.44	4.30	4.19	4.10	3.96	3.82	3.66	3.59	3.51	3.43	3.34	3.25	3.17
14	8.86	6.51	5.56	5.04	4.69	4.46	4.28	4.14	4.03	3.94	3.80	3.66	3.51	3.43	3.35	3.27	3.18	3.09	3.00
15	8.68	6.36	5.42	4.89	4.56	4.32	4.14	4.00	3.89	3.80	3.67	3.52	3.37	3.29	3.21	3.13	3.05	2.96	2.87
16	8.53	6.23	5.29	4.77	4.44	4.20	4.03	3.89	3.78	3.69	3.55	3.41	3.26	3.18	3.10	3.02	2.93	2.84	2.75
17	8.40	6.11	5.18	4.67	4.34	4.10	3.93	3.79	3.68	3.59	3.46	3.31	3.16	3.08	3.00	2.92	2.83	2.75	2.65
18	8.29	6.01	5.09	4.58	4.25	4.01	3.84	3.71	3.60	3.51	3.37	3.23	3.08	3.00	2.92	2.84	2.75	2.66	2.57
19	8.18	5.93	5.01	4.50	4.17	3.94	3.77	3.63	3.52	3.43	3.30	3.15	3.00	2.92	2.84	2.76	2.67	2.58	2.49
20	8.10	5.85	4.94	4.43	4.10	3.87	3.70	3.56	3.46	3.37	3.23	3.09	2.94	2.86	2.78	2.69	2.61	2.52	2.42
21	8.02	5.78	4.87	4.37	4.04	3.81	3.64	3.51	3.40	3.31	3.17	3.03	2.88	2.80	2.72	2.64	2.55	2.46	2.36
22	7.95	5.72	4.82	4.31	3.99	3.76	3.59	3.45	3.35	3.26	3.12	2.98	2.83	2.75	2.67	2.58	2.50	2.40	2.31
23	7.88	5.66	4.76	4.26	3.94	3.71	3.54	3.41	3.30	3.21	3.07	2.93	2.78	2.70	2.62	2.54	2.45	2.35	2.26
24	7.82	5.61	4.72	4.22	3.90	3.67	3.50	3.36	3.26	3.17	3.03	2.89	2.74	2.66	2.58	2.49	2.40	2.31	2.21
25	7.77	5.57	4.68	4.18	3.85	3.63	3.46	3.32	3.22	3.13	2.99	2.85	2.70	2.62	2.54	2.45	2.36	2.27	2.17
26	7.72	5.53	4.64	4.14	3.82	3.59	3.42	3.29	3.18	3.09	2.96	2.81	2.66	2.58	2.50	2.42	2.33	2.23	2.13
27	7.68	5.49	4.60	4.11	3.78	3.56	3.39	3.26	3.15	3.06	2.93	2.78	2.63	2.55	2.47	2.38	2.29	2.20	2.10
28	7.64	5.45	4.57	4.07	3.75	3.53	3.36	3.23	3.12	3.03	2.90	2.75	2.60	2.52	2.44	2.35	2.26	2.17	2.06
29	7.60	5.42	4.54	4.04	3.73	3.50	3.33	3.20	3.09	3.00	2.87	2.73	2.57	2.49	2.41	2.33	2.23	2.14	2.03
30	7.56	5.39	4.51	4.02	3.70	3.47	3.30	3.17	3.07	2.98	2.84	2.70	2.55	2.47	2.39	2.30	2.21	2.11	2.01
40	7.31	5.18	4.31	3.83	3.51	3.29	3.12	2.99	2.89	2.80	2.66	2.52	2.37	2.29	2.20	2.11	2.02	1.92	1.80
60	7.08	4.98	4.13	3.65	3.34	3.12	2.95	2.82	2.72	2.63	2.50	2.35	2.20	2.12	2.03	1.94	1.84	1.73	1.60
120	6.85	4.79	3.95	3.48	3.17	2.96	2.79	2.66	2.56	2.47	2.34	2.19	2.03	1.95	1.86	1.76	1.66	1.53	1.38
∞	6.63	4.61	3.78	3.32	3.02	2.80	2.64	2.51	2.41	2.32	2.18	2.04	1.88	1.79	1.70	1.59	1.47	1.32	1.00

V_1, V_2, are upper, lower d.f. respectively.

Table 5 The Studentized Range, Q $p = 0.05$

Degrees of Freedom	Number of Treatments																		
	2	3	4	5	6	7	8	9	10	11	12	13	14	15	16	17	18	19	20
1	18.0	27.0	32.8	37.2	40.5	43.1	45.4	47.3	49.1	50.6	51.9	53.2	54.3	55.4	56.3	57.2	58.0	58.8	59.6
2	6.09	8.33	9.80	10.89	11.73	12.43	13.03	13.54	13.99	14.39	14.75	15.08	15.38	15.65	15.91	16.14	16.36	16.57	16.77
3	4.50	5.91	6.83	7.51	8.04	8.47	8.85	9.18	9.46	9.72	9.95	10.16	10.35	10.52	10.69	10.84	10.98	11.12	11.24
4	3.93	5.04	5.76	6.29	6.71	7.06	7.35	7.60	7.83	8.03	8.21	8.37	8.52	8.67	8.80	8.92	9.03	9.14	9.24
5	3.64	4.60	5.22	5.67	6.03	6.33	6.58	6.80	6.99	7.17	7.32	7.47	7.60	7.72	7.83	7.93	8.03	8.12	8.21
6	3.46	4.34	4.90	5.31	5.63	5.89	6.12	6.32	6.49	6.65	6.79	6.92	7.04	7.14	7.24	7.34	7.43	7.51	7.59
7	3.34	4.16	4.68	5.06	5.35	5.59	5.80	5.99	6.15	6.29	6.42	6.54	6.65	6.75	6.84	6.93	7.01	7.08	7.16
8	3.26	4.04	4.53	4.89	5.17	5.40	5.60	5.77	5.92	6.05	6.18	6.29	6.39	6.48	6.57	6.65	6.73	6.80	6.87
9	3.20	3.95	4.42	4.76	5.02	5.24	5.43	5.60	5.74	5.87	5.98	6.09	6.19	6.28	6.36	6.44	6.51	6.58	6.65
10	3.15	3.88	4.33	4.66	4.91	5.12	5.30	5.46	5.60	5.72	5.83	5.93	6.03	6.12	6.20	6.27	6.34	6.41	6.47
11	3.11	3.82	4.26	4.58	4.82	5.03	5.20	5.35	5.49	5.61	5.71	5.81	5.90	5.98	6.06	6.14	6.20	6.27	6.33
12	3.08	3.77	4.20	4.51	4.75	4.95	5.12	5.27	5.40	5.51	5.61	5.71	5.80	5.88	5.95	6.02	6.09	6.15	6.21
13	3.06	3.73	4.15	4.46	4.69	4.88	5.05	5.19	5.32	5.43	5.53	5.63	5.71	5.79	5.86	5.93	6.00	6.06	6.11
14	3.03	3.70	4.11	4.41	4.64	4.83	4.99	5.13	5.25	5.36	5.46	5.56	5.64	5.72	5.79	5.86	5.92	5.98	6.03
15	3.01	3.67	4.08	4.37	4.59	4.78	4.94	5.08	5.20	5.31	5.40	5.49	5.57	5.65	5.72	5.79	5.85	5.91	5.96
16	3.00	3.65	4.05	4.34	4.56	4.74	4.90	5.03	5.15	5.26	5.35	5.44	5.52	5.59	5.66	5.73	5.79	5.84	5.90
17	2.98	3.62	4.02	4.31	4.52	4.70	4.86	4.99	5.11	5.21	5.31	5.39	5.47	5.55	5.61	5.68	5.74	5.79	5.84
18	2.97	3.61	4.00	4.28	4.49	4.67	4.83	4.96	5.07	5.17	5.27	5.35	5.43	5.50	5.57	5.63	5.69	5.74	5.79
19	2.96	3.59	3.98	4.26	4.47	4.64	4.79	4.92	5.04	5.14	5.23	5.32	5.39	5.46	5.53	5.59	5.65	5.70	5.75
20	2.95	3.58	3.96	4.24	4.45	4.62	4.77	4.90	5.01	5.11	5.20	5.28	5.36	5.43	5.50	5.56	5.61	5.66	5.71
24	2.92	3.53	3.90	4.17	4.37	4.54	4.68	4.81	4.92	5.01	5.10	5.18	5.25	5.32	5.38	5.44	5.50	5.55	5.59
30	2.89	3.48	3.84	4.11	4.30	4.46	4.60	4.72	4.83	4.92	5.00	5.08	5.15	5.21	5.27	5.33	5.38	5.43	5.48
40	2.86	3.44	3.79	4.04	4.23	4.39	4.52	4.63	4.74	4.82	4.90	4.98	5.05	5.11	5.17	5.22	5.27	5.32	5.36
60	2.83	3.40	3.74	3.98	4.16	4.31	4.44	4.55	4.65	4.73	4.81	4.88	4.94	5.00	5.06	5.11	5.15	5.20	5.24
120	2.80	3.36	3.69	3.92	4.10	4.24	4.36	4.47	4.56	4.64	4.71	4.78	4.84	4.90	4.95	5.00	5.04	5.09	5.13
∞	2.77	3.32	3.63	3.86	4.03	4.17	4.29	4.39	4.47	4.55	4.62	4.68	4.74	4.80	4.84	4.89	4.93	4.97	5.01

(Reproduced with permission, from Table A15 of SNEDECOR and COCHRANE: *Statistical Methods*, 6th edn. (1967), Iowa State University Press)

Table 6 Critical values of F_{max} p = 0.05 (upper), p = 0.01 (lower).

n−1 \ k	2	3	4	5	6	7	8	9	10	11	12
2	39.0 / 199.	87.5 / 448.	142. / 729.	202. / 1036	266. / 1362	333. / 1705	403. / 2063	475. / 2432	550. / 2813	626. / 3204	704. / 3605
3	15.4 / 47.5	27.8 / 85.	39.2 / 120.	50.7 / 151.	62.0 / 184.	72.9 / 216(.)	83.5 / 249(.)	93.9 / 281(.)	104 / 310(.)	114. / 337(.)	124. / 361(.)
4	9.60 / 23.2	15.5 / 37.	20.6 / 49.	25.2 / 59.	29.5 / 69.	33.6 / 79.	37.5 / 89.	41.1 / 97.	44.6 / 106.	48.0 / 113.	51.4 / 120.
5	7.15 / 14.9	10.8 / 22.	13.7 / 28.	16.3 / 33.	18.7 / 38.	20.8 / 42.	22.9 / 46.	24.7 / 50.	26.5 / 54.	28.2 / 57.	29.9 / 60.
6	5.82 / 11.1	8.38 / 15.5	10.4 / 19.1	12.1 / 22.	13.7 / 25.	15.0 / 27.	16.3 / 30.	17.5 / 32.	18.6 / 34.	19.7 / 36.	20.7 / 37.
7	4.99 / 8.89	6.94 / 12.1	8.44 / 14.5	9.70 / 16.5	10.8 / 18.4	11.8 / 20.	12.7 / 22.	13.5 / 23.	14.3 / 24.	15.1 / 26.	15.8 / 27.
8	4.43 / 7.50	6.00 / 9.9	7.18 / 11.7	8.12 / 13.2	9.03 / 14.5	9.78 / 15.8	10.5 / 16.9	11.1 / 17.9	11.7 / 18.9	12.2 / 19.8	12.7 / 21.
9	4.03 / 6.54	5.34 / 8.5	6.31 / 9.9	7.11 / 11.1	7.80 / 12.1	8.41 / 13.1	8.95 / 13.9	9.45 / 14.7	9.91 / 15.3	10.3 / 16.0	10.7 / 16.6
10	3.72 / 5.85	4.85 / 7.4	5.67 / 8.6	6.34 / 9.6	6.92 / 10.4	7.42 / 11.1	7.87 / 11.8	8.28 / 12.4	8.66 / 12.9	9.01 / 13.4	9.34 / 13.9
12	3.28 / 4.91	4.16 / 6.1	4.75 / 6.9	5.30 / 7.6	5.72 / 8.2	6.09 / 8.7	6.42 / 9.1	6.72 / 9.5	7.00 / 9.9	7.25 / 10.2	7.43 / 10.6
15	2.86 / 4.07	3.54 / 4.9	4.01 / 5.5	4.37 / 6.0	4.68 / 6.4	4.95 / 6.7	5.19 / 7.1	5.40 / 7.3	5.59 / 7.5	5.77 / 7.8	5.93 / 8.0
20	2.46 / 3.32	2.95 / 3.8	3.29 / 4.3	3.54 / 4.6	3.76 / 4.9	3.94 / 5.1	4.10 / 5.3	4.24 / 5.5	4.37 / 5.6	4.49 / 5.8	4.59 / 5.9
30	2.07 / 2.63	2.40 / 3.0	2.61 / 3.3	2.78 / 3.4	2.91 / 3.6	3.02 / 3.7	3.12 / 3.8	3.21 / 3.9	3.29 / 4.0	3.36 / 4.1	3.39 / 4.2
60	1.67 / 1.96	1.85 / 2.2	1.96 / 2.3	2.04 / 2.4	2.11 / 2.4	2.17 / 2.5	2.22 / 2.5	2.26 / 2.6	2.30 / 2.6	2.33 / 2.7	2.36 / 2.7
∞	1.00 / 1.00	1.00 / 1.0	1.00 / 1.0	1.00 / 1.0	1.00 / 1.0	1.00 / 1.0	1.00 / 1.0	1.00 / 1.0	1.00 / 1.0	1.00 / 1.0	1.00 / 1.0